New Paradigms in Healthcare

In the first two decades of this new millennium, the self-sufficiency of Evidence-Based Medicine (EBM) have begun to be questioned. The narrative version gradually assumed increasing importance as the need emerged to shift to more biologically, psychologically, socially, and existentially focused models. The terrible experience of the COVID pandemic truly revealed that EBM alone, while being a wonderful scientific philosophy and containing the physician's paternalistic approach, has its limitations: it often ignores both the patient's and physician's perspectives as persons, as human beings; it pays relentless attention to biological markers and not to the more personal, psychological, social, and anthropological ones, removing the emotions, thoughts, and desires of life, focusing on just the "measurable quality" of it.

Health Humanities, Medical Humanities and Narrative Medicine are arts intertwined with sciences that allow to broaden the mindset and approach of healthcare professionals. helping them to produce better care and more well-being.

Aim of this series is to collect "person-centered" contributions, as only a multidisciplinary and collaborative team can meet the challenge of combining the multiple aspects of human health, as well as the health of our planet, and of all the creatures that live on it, in a common effort to stop or reverse the enormous damage committed by humans during our anthropocentric era: a new paradigm of healthcare, education and learning to create a sustainable health system.

Sabina Leoncini

The Relationship between Pharmacists and Patients

Care and Complexity

Springer

Sabina Leoncini
Department of Political and Cognitive Sciences
University of Siena
Siena, Italy

ISSN 2731-3247 ISSN 2731-3255 (electronic)
New Paradigms in Healthcare
ISBN 978-3-032-21248-1 ISBN 978-3-032-21249-8 (eBook)
https://doi.org/10.1007/978-3-032-21249-8

This Springer imprint is published by the registered company Springer Nature Switzerland AG
The registered company address is: Gewerbestrasse 11, 6330 Cham, Switzerland

Foreword

The realization of this monograph is driven by a deep conviction: The pharmaceutical profession, far from being a static and purely technical practice, is undergoing a profound transformation, positioning itself at the intersection of scientific rigor, technological innovation, and the complexity of care. The creation of this text, in fact, as is evident from its internal structure, is guided by the desire to move beyond the image of the pharmacist as a mere dispenser of medicines, and to rediscover their more complete identity as a caregiver and a relational mediator in support of social cohesion and health equity.

The exploration proposed by the work begins with a historical perspective that serves as an essential return to the origins (Chap. 1). The discussion of the evolution of the pharmacist's role, from the Egyptians and Greeks (Hippocrates) up to Roman influence (Galen) and the Salerno School, does not merely have an academic value, but constitutes the necessary anchor for appreciating the scientific solidity of the discipline. This historical analysis, as the reader will discover, will help them understand and define the boundaries of medical and pharmaceutical science and appreciate how the present is the product of a millennial tradition of research and practice.

Continuing this exploration, the author highlights that the proposed idea of care is fueled and supported by values such as listening, dialogue, and empathy (Chap. 2), which give the professional the ability to intervene in unexpected situations. It is in this dimension, which involves not only the body but also the deep meanings of the illness experience, that I believe the pharmacist finds their deepest *raison d'être*; the reflection on the right to care meets the right to illness and dignity, reminding us that assistance is not only a medical matter but an ethical imperative of respect, listening, and nondiscrimination.

But there is more that can serve the reader of this work, and which emerges clearly as we delve into its pages. The sense of care discussed cannot ignore the systemic realities that shape or limit this concept. Understanding the profound structural inequalities that generate the "poverty of care," often deny equitable access to healthcare and amplify social and economic disparities (Chap. 3), implicitly strengthens the idea that the pharmacist is a relational mediator whose task is twofold: to combat stereotypes and prejudices and act concretely for the promotion of health equity.

If this is the case, the care of others then appears inseparable from self-care (Chap. 4), and to provide empathetic and sustainable assistance, the pharmacist must, in turn, bc a subject who is cared for. Autobiographical writing, psychosocial development, well-being linked to beauty, and, above all, burn-out among healthcare workers have become an opportunity to reaffirm this principle and remind us that *cura sui* (care of self) is an ethical as much as transformative practice.

These considerations find a crucial testing ground in the central part of this work through the exploration of a specific Italian case study (Chap. 5), which allows the reader (especially those at the beginning of their professional career) to connect the text to a formative dimension of "learning by doing." The example of rural pharmacies, essential for territorial cohesion, the impact of educational reforms, and the direct testimonies of psychologists and pharmacists that are reported, as well as the application of the narrative medicine approach to the pharmacist profession, confirm that the transformation is already underway and see this professional as an essential relational mediator.

Following this perspective, the chapter concerning the medical humanities (Chap. 6) is not to be considered an appendix, but represents a strong theoretical framework (which the author of the work decided to reveal, preserving the anticipation, almost at the end of the text) that holds together what the reader has learned and discussed up to that point. The integration of evidence-based medicine with narrative-based approaches allows one to overcome the limits of the biomedical model, placing the patient's lived experience at the center of the therapeutic path. The conviction that narrative can become a tool for healing and identity reconstruction, thus, provides further scope for intervention for the ethics of care that has been discussed and consistently supports the epistemological challenge posed by this approach.

Having reached the end of the text, the reader is implicitly confronted with a question that perhaps they have preserved throughout the reading of the work: What can be the future of this professional today (Chap. 7), who is asked to be the "custodian of care" but also, simultaneously, to rely on digital technologies and AI? The challenge of the future, for which the work intelligently reserves space for analysis, proposes a balanced approach where technology is a *complement* and not a *substitute* for human care. This is why the pharmacist again assumes the figure of a complex professional: One who embraces digital literacy and AI, but does so with an ethical compass firmly oriented toward professional responsibility and patient trust.

Ultimately, this monograph appears to me as an important invitation to view the pharmacist not only as a technician expert in medicines but as a custodian of care in a complex perspective: A figure who combines the scientific competence inherited from a millennial history with the emotional and narrative intelligence required by our present and future. It is in this dynamic synthesis—between pharmacy as an exact science and pharmacy as a relational art—that the profession can fully fulfill its vital role. A role that is more crucial than ever in a society marked by profound contradictions, ideological polarizations, and a growing tendency toward the trivialization of thought and action.

Carlo Orefice
Associate Professor of General and Social Pedagogy at the University of Siena
Florence, Italy
October 3, 2025

Preface

The history of pharmacy mirrors humanity's long-standing effort to give structure, meaning, and method to the act of caring. From the magical remedies of ancient civilizations to the more complex medical systems developed by Egyptians, Chinese, Sumerians, Indians, and Incas, human beings have progressively shaped a pharmaceutical knowledge that, through Greek and Roman contributions, monastic traditions, the advances of the Islamic world, and major medieval reforms, eventually acquired a stable institutional and professional form in Europe. This millenary trajectory is not only technical; it also expresses humanity's enduring tension toward taking care of oneself and others—an aspiration that today translates into the pharmacist as a healthcare professional, cultural mediator, and social actor.

Care extends well beyond its clinical dimension. It is a relational, communicative, and deeply human phenomenon. It involves listening, empathy, dialogue, and the capacity to navigate uncertainty. In the pharmacist's daily work, care emerges in the ability to respond to the unexpected, build meaningful relationships, and accompany people through vulnerable experiences. This broader view is essential in a world marked by profound socioeconomic and cultural disparities.

Recent global crises, including the COVID-19 pandemic, have shown how biological vulnerabilities intersect with social ones, revealing the syndemic nature of contemporary health challenges. In this context, pharmacists serve as key agents of health equity: not only providers of therapies, but also professionals capable of counteracting stereotypes, prejudice, and cultural barriers. Adopting biopsychosocial approaches redefines the pharmacy as a relational space in which understanding the patient's lived experience becomes integral to therapeutic practice. Psychological phenomena, such as the influence of expectations on patient motivation and adherence, further underscore the ethical responsibility embedded in pharmaceutical care.

The theme of care intersects with that of self-care, a concept with ancient roots stretching from classical philosophy to contemporary interpretations. Self-care emerges as a continuous process of personal development, responsibility, and relational awareness. It concerns identity, emotional regulation, and the ability to construct one's own narrative. Within pharmaceutical practice, this includes attention to psychological aspects of health—from the relationship individuals maintain with their bodies, visible, for instance, in cosmetic practices from antiquity to modern clinical use, to the vulnerability associated with psychoactive substance use in performance-driven societies. At the same time, the rise of burn-out among healthcare professionals, including pharmacists, highlights the need for systemic interventions that safeguard well-being and ensure the safe, effective delivery of care.

These dynamics gain particular significance in the Italian context, where over 7200 rural pharmacies represent the main, and often only, healthcare access point for millions of citizens. Recent reforms—ranging from economic support and hybrid remuneration models to digital innovation and new educational pathways with direct professional qualification—acknowledge the strategic role of pharmacists in territorial cohesion and public health. Interviews and qualitative studies reveal a transforming professional identity increasingly defined by relational, narrative, and humanistic dimensions. The pharmacist is progressively understood not only as a dispenser of medicines but also as a listener and interpreter of patient stories, working within interdisciplinary teams and fostering trust through communication and empathy.

Within this perspective, the medical humanities offer a conceptual and practical framework that reconnects technological and scientific knowledge with the human experience of illness. Narrative medicine, and more specifically narrative pharmacy, emphasize the interpretive value of stories—those of patients as well as those shared among professionals. This approach aims to humanize care, strengthen therapeutic alliances, and acknowledge the emotional and symbolic dimensions of health and illness. In the aftermath of widespread institutional distrust and social fragmentation, narrative and relational approaches help rebuild trust and encourage active citizen participation in health decision-making.

The volume also explores the relationship between pharmacy and alternative epistemological models, such as homeopathy, phytotherapy, and naturopathy. These traditions propose a vitalistic and holistic understanding of health that emphasizes systemic balance and the body's self-regulatory capacities. While they pose an epistemic challenge to biomedical paradigms, they converge with humanistic approaches in promoting care as education, participation, and reconnection with the natural world.

The final chapter looks toward the future. Digital innovation—through online pharmacies, telepharmacy, and artificial intelligence—is reshaping pharmaceutical practice and healthcare delivery. These technologies offer new opportunities for accessibility, personalization, and efficiency, yet also raise concerns related to counterfeit medicines, data protection, and the erosion of human relationships. The pharmacist of the future will need strong digital literacy, ethical sensitivity, and the ability to integrate technological tools without compromising the relational core of care. Ultimately, the challenge lies in ensuring that innovation complements, rather than replaces, the human dimensions that define the profession.

This volume, thus, proposes a broad, interdisciplinary, and profoundly humanistic vision of pharmacy: a profession rooted in a millenary history and called today to redefine itself at the intersection of science and narrative, technique and relationship, individual and community, technology and humanity.

Siena, Italy
Sabina Leoncini

Acknowledgments

The genesis of this book is connected to, on the one hand, personal reasons and, on the other, scholarly curiosity. I thank my father; his tenacity in facing his illness gave me the courage to approach the topic of care from many different perspectives.

The scholarly origin of this book is linked to the establishment of the course "The Complexity of the Pharmacist–Patient Relationship: Toward a Pedagogy of Care," offered for the first time within the Degree Programme in Pharmacy at the University of Siena. I wish to thank Professor Sandra Gemma and Professor Antonella Brizzi for their warm welcome and for organizing the course. I am grateful to Professor Carlo Orefice and Professor Maria Rita Mancaniello, my mentor, for guiding me through the construction of the syllabus and reinforcing my conviction that courses of this kind should be available in all universities.

I am deeply grateful to all the students enrolled in the Degree Programme in Pharmacy who attended the course during the 2024–2025 academic year, as well as those who participated in 2025–2026. Their contributions—through reflections, discussions and focus groups—enabled me to develop a pedagogical pathway grounded in student feedback and oriented toward a dialogical co-construction of knowledge. The contribution of Maria Ernestina Faggiano and Daniela Scala from SIFO, as well as that of a psychologist working in the oncology department of an Italian hospital, whose name I omit for privacy reasons, were equally important.

I would also like to thank Giancarlo Signore and Tito Piccioni for letting me visit the historic headquarters of the Nobile Collegio Chimico Farmaceutico at Via in Miranda 10, in Rome, from which you can admire the beauty of the Roman Forum, and let me breathe in the centuries of history this place has spanned.

Thanks to Philip Saunders for accompanying me throughout the proofreading process, which he followed with great dedication.

Naturally, I would not have been able to write this book without the support of my family, who have always stood by me, even during moments of fatigue and stress, to which everyday life relentlessly subjects us. Finally, my deepest gratitude goes to Springer, and in particular to Maria Giulia Marini and Jonathan McFarland, who believed in this project from the outset and placed their trust in me.

Contents

Chapter 1
The Role of the Pharmacist: A Historical Perspective on the Birth and Evolution of the Pharmacist

1.1 Introduction

Stéphane Laurent emerges in the recent volume (2025), *The Doctor and the Shaman: Dialogue on the Cure and Healing* by Artur and Stéphane Laurent [1], in my opinion, as the emblem of the dilemma that has always distressed man. After having dedicated his life to pharmacological research, the established Parisian cardiologist Stéphane Laurent, decides to question his scientific beliefs to confront his son Artur, an apprentice shaman in an indigenous community in the Amazon. The phenomenon of shamanism has been witnessed by historians, ethnologists and sociologists of religions in tens of thousands of different tribes around the world, from Siberia to the Amazon, from the Alps to the Andes. From the exchange of ideas between father (Stéphane) and son (Artur), the reader can discover shamanic healing rituals: songs, energy flows, master plants and, above all, *Ayahuasca*, an infusion with powerful hallucinogenic effects capable of generating altered states of consciousness. Without underestimating the risks associated with its intake, the author explores the surprising pharmacological properties of this drink, which could offer new therapeutic possibilities for neuropsychological disorders that are still difficult to treat, such as depression, anxiety, post-traumatic stress and chronic pain. Man has always wondered how to cure body and soul. On the one hand, there are supporters of conventional medicine, and on the other, there are enthusiasts of alternative medicine. What they have in common is the need to rethink their concept of care, health and well-being, which is also the aim of my book, which begins with another story, the history of the pharmacy.

S. Leoncini, *The Relationship between Pharmacists and Patients*, New Paradigms in Healthcare, https://doi.org/10.1007/978-3-032-21249-8_1

1.2 At the Dawn of Human Civilization: The Practice of Healing Emerges from the Ice

The Tyrolean Iceman Ötzi is the world's oldest glacier mummy. He was found in the Ötztal Alps in September 1991. Since his discovery, a variety of morphological, radiological and molecular analyses have been performed that revealed detailed insights into his state of health. Despite the various pathological conditions found in the Iceman, little is known about possible forms of care and treatment during the Copper Age in this area [2]. A possible approach to this topic is the presence of tattoos on the mummified body. In previous work, it was already believed that the tattoos were administered as a kind of treatment for his lower back pain and degenerative joint disease of his knees, hip and wrist. In other studies, the tattoos of the Iceman have been related to an early form of acupuncture [3]. The researchers evaluated the various health issues of the Iceman, including joint diseases, gastrointestinal problems and arterial calcifications, and compared them to the location and number of tattoos. Together with the finding of medically effective fungi and plants, such as the birch polypore or fern in his equipment and intestines, the researchers suggested that care and treatment was already common during the Iceman's time.

1.3 The Golden Bough

Before setting out on his journey to the realm of the dead, Aeneas picked the golden bough at the Sibyl's invitation. According to the ancients, this legend was linked to the strange custom whereby only those who managed to tear off a branch from the tree that grew in the enclosure of Diana's sanctuary at Nemi, killing the priest who watched over those places, could succeed as *king of the woods*. Struck by what seemed to be a barbaric custom that had survived up to imperial times, James Frazer embarked on a search for the universal motifs that could have inspired it, comparing myths and rites from every time and place. James G. Frazer (1854–1941) is one of the "founding fathers" of social anthropology, a discipline in which he held the first chair in the world in Liverpool in 1908. His research ranged from classical and biblical cultures to primitive ones, producing work that, in addition to *The Golden Bough* [4], includes *Totemism and Exogamy* [5], *Folk-Lore in the Old Testament* [6] and *The Magical Origin of Kings* [7]. An obligatory point of reference for ethnologists and anthropologists, Frazer is also considered one of the greatest writers of his time. In many moments of his book, such as the one cited here, he recounts rituals on the border between magic and religion that, although belonging to different cultures and various eras, resemble each other and have analogies despite their protagonists never having met.

> Another beneficial use of homeopathic magic is to cure or prevent disease. The ancient Hindus performed an elaborate ceremony based on homeopathic magic for the treatment of jaundice. Its main purpose was to pass the color yellow to yellow creatures and

things (such as the sun) to which it rightfully belongs, and to procure for the patient the color red of health, from a living and vigorous source, namely a red bull. With this intention, a priest recited the following words of a magical nature: "To the sun may your heartache and your jaundice ascend; in the color of the red bull we envelop you! We envelop you in the color red for a long life. May this person emerge unharmed and free from the color yellow. In the cows, whose deity is Rohini, and who are also red (rohinih) themselves, in all their forms and all their strengths we envelop you! In the parrots and in the thrushes we put your jaundice; in the yellow wagtail we put your jaundice again." And while he was pronouncing these words, in order to infuse the rosy color of health into the pale patient, the priest gave him to drink water with the hairs of a red bull in it; he poured water on the animal's back and made the patient drink it; he made him sit on the skin of a red bull and tied a piece of it to his body. To improve therefore his color, and to completely drive away the yellow tint, he proceeded as follows. He first smeared him from head to foot with a yellow paste made of saffron or turmeric (a yellow plant); he laid him on a bed, and tied with a yellow ribbon to the foot of the bed three yellow birds, namely a parrot, a thrush, and a yellow wagtail; then, pouring water over the patient, he washed away the yellow mush, and no doubt also the jaundice with it, which was transferred to the three birds. After that, in order to make his complexion completely bloom, he took some of the hair of a red bull, wrapped it in gold leaf, and stuck it on the skin of his patient. The ancients believed that if a patient with jaundice were to look fixedly at a woodcock, and the bird looked at him, he would be cured of his disease. "Such is the nature," says Plutarch, "such is the temperament of this animal that it extracts and receives into itself the disease, which passes like a current through the glance." This precious property of the woodcock was so well recognized among bird dealers that when they had one of these birds to sell, they kept it carefully covered, so that a jaundice patient would not look at it and would be treated for free. ([4] p. 39)

1.4 The History of Human Beings

Human beings lived as nomads by moving from one place to another, and then started to allocate and expand their land by integrating their diet with meat and fish. The first form of care that we can trace through archaeological and anthropological studies is prayer and hope. Some ethnologists believe that magic and religion have been generated to escape the fear and mystery that impinged into the life of primitive man. Particularly the Magi not only in the ancient Persian religion but also Babylonian are astrologers, fortune tellers and sorcerers. They were then called kings in the Gospels of the New Testament who were led by a star to come to Bethlehem to pay homage to the baby Jesus. Magic was certainly a prodrome of science and research; also religion, in the case of Islam, since the ninth century CE. It extended knowledge and promoted a great impulse to philosophical studies, and mathematical and astronomical sciences, in addition to medical-pharmaceutical research. Other religions, due to the priestly caste, were an obstacle to social and scientific progress. What still appears surprising today is the fact that several peoples in different areas of the world (India, China, Egypt, Greece), without any contact to each other, used medications based on very similar herbs to treat equally similar diseases in the same historical period.

1.5 The Egyptians

The medical knowledge of the Egyptians was highly appreciated throughout the Near East and also among the Greeks, so much so that Herodotus wrote in his stories that "there are doctors everywhere" in Egypt. He tells of periods of fasting in which laxatives were taken, such as dates, tamarinds or senna pulp infusions. Even nowadays, scholars, such as Hans-W. Fischer-Elfert, study the medical treaties found in Egyptian papyri that explain the use of cosmetics contained in particular vessels that also had the intention of treating eye diseases. Homer, for his part, claims in *The Odyssey* that Egypt is the land where doctors overcome all other men in skill, so much so that Elena brought a miraculous drug from there called nepenthe to Sparta, which calmed anger and pain, oblivious of all penalties [8]. Around the end of the nineteenth century, the first Egyptian papyri dating back to 2000 BCE were discovered by Edward Smith, Giorgio Von Ebers and Giuseppe Passalacqua. In particular, the second (dating to about 1700 BCE) is even defined as the first "pharmacopoeia" understood as "drug-to-party", which, thus, describes the art of preparing the drug. There are testimonies of finding tombs containing iron and opium, which were prescribed as medicines with medicinal herbs. However, we should not criticize the Egyptian pharmacopoeia, but grasp its constructive aspects. In fact, the miraculous recipes were written as part of the subject of study of the medical toothbrush. One can glean from this the fact that the Egyptians were a very healthy people whose scholars observed the cause and effect regarding the medical advice that was given. The practice of using an enema, for example, was discovered by the ancient Egyptians. Putting the body was one of the essential therapeutic intentions of the Egyptian doctor and it was also so in other civilizations for Hippocrates and Galenic-Arab medicine.

1.6 The Chinese

The origin of acupuncture is lost in the mists of legendary times, in which the fight against disease was a fight against evil spirits [9, 10]. Traces of this still remain in the modern energetic structure of acupuncture in the name of a form of acupuncture called "Thirteen Demons". There are some explanations concerning the discovery of acupuncture that derive the beginnings of this practice from shamanic rituals in which the insertion of needles would have had the function of chasing away or killing the "evil spirits" that, having taken possession of a man and located themselves in certain places, caused the disease. The use of acupuncture in an apotropaic sense can probably be traced back to the Neolithic period (8000–5000 BCE). In this period, the acupuncture points were probably stimulated with sharp stone splinters or other easily available materials, such as bone splinters or bamboo, as some archaeological finds testify. However, the historical birth of acupuncture, as it is known today, is difficult to date and we find it more as a consolidated practice, provided with a robust theoretical apparatus, than as an empirical fact "in progress" that structures its theory as experience is enriched. Some classical texts and a series of information obtainable from finds from various archaeological sites testify that the history of acupuncture probably began with the Shang dynasty (1600–1100 BCE). In this period, needles made of bronze, copper, tin, gold or silver were already available. It is probable, however, that older materials were still used for acupuncture, such as thorns from different plants, bamboo splinters, bone, horn or jade. Numerous schools of thought were born during the Warring States period (475–221 BCE): Concerning the Taoist School, TCM regards the concept of *Tao* as a law determining all natural phenomena and that of *Qi* as an energy ascertaining the origin and maintenance of being. In the Taoist conception, medicine and its techniques (e.g. acupuncture, dietetics, pharmacology, breathing exercises and meditation) were at the service of the sage in his journey towards sainthood. We owe the theory of the same name to the Naturalistic School or School of Yin-Yang as a method for knowing and interpreting reality. The Confucian School then introduced the concepts of "Order" and "Model", establishing a hierarchy of organs and viscera, organized in a similar way to the hierarchy of the state. Three fundamental texts were written: one of applied pharmacology, the *Shennong Bencao Jing*; one of diagnosis and therapy, the *Treatise on Febrile and Mixed Diseases* (written by the famous doctor Zhang Zhong Jing, who emphasizes, for the first time, the usefulness of the association of acupuncture with pharmacotherapy); and the last, the *Classic of Acupuncture and Moxibustion*. In the latter, you can find the location and indications of 649 acupuncture points, and it also constitutes a complete treatment of the theory and practice of acupuncture-moxibustion, including contraindications. The author Huangfu Mi (214–282 CE) wrote this text by sifting and reorganizing all the material on acupuncture present in the *Medical Classic of the Yellow Emperor*.

1.7 The Incas, Sumerians and Indians

The Incas had some specific ideas about the pathogenesis and course of a disease which were completely different from the modern Western view of medicine [11]. These ideas are essential for the understanding of Inca medicine in general and the role of the healer in particular. They are the reason that the Spanish chroniclers often wrote in a negative sense about the medical practitioners of Peru. While the profound knowledge of medicinal plants was experienced by the Spaniards as a positive feature, the large and intimate involvement of religion and magic in Inca medicine and its practitioners was a feature that did not contribute to its popularity among the Western invaders. For the Incas, a close relationship existed between religion and magic on the one hand, and disease on the other. Disease was seen as the result of a disturbed relationship with supernatural forces. The Sumerians documented the first collection of healing substances, as well as pharmaceutical formulas and indications about their preparation, which was identified on a tablet found in

Nippur and dated 2300 BCE. *Ayurveda* (science of life) and *Atharveda* (science of magic formulas) treatises from ancient India are among the written evidence and sacred books. Ayurveda is referred directly to the creator god Brahma, who transmitted the secret of getting rid of diseases causing harm to living beings. It deals with the relationship between man and nature; the spirit, human body and surrounding environment are seen as a whole; therefore, it is necessary to assess and heal the entire system to regain well-being and health. The *Atharvaveda* includes medical thoughts inspired by magic with the use of vegetable drugs; one thousand of them were listed, many of which have also been widely used during the succeeding centuries.

1.8 The Greeks

The word *phármakon* referred to both toxic substances and medications in ancient Greece. Medications were considered to be substances aimed at treating a disease. During the fourth century BCE, Hippocrates asserted that drugs are all those substances that are able to change the existing condition of the body or determine its functional change. This definition of a drug, which does not differentiate between a potentially harmful substance and one that may provide benefit to a sick person, is still in use. Nowadays, the word "drug" refers to any substance that determines functional changes in the body, used for treatment purposes or to understand the physiological processes and the diagnosis of diseases. Therefore, it includes the contrast systems used in a magnetic resonance imaging. The definition of a drug given by the World Health Organization (WHO) agrees with this statement: "any chemical substance or product used to modify or examine physiological functions or pathological conditions to the benefit of patients" [12].

> Sing, O goddess, the anger of Achilles son of Peleus, that brought countless ills upon the Achaeans. Many a brave soul did it send hurrying down to Hades, and many a hero did it yield a prey to dogs and vultures, for so were the counsels of Jove fulfilled from the day on which the son of Atreus, king of men, and great Achilles, first fell out with one another.
>
> And which of the gods was it that set them on to quarrel. It was the son of Jove and Leto; for he was angry with the king and sent a pestilence upon the host to plague the people, because the son of Atreus had dishonoured Chryses his priest. Now Chryses had come to the ships of the Achseans to free his daughter, and had brought with him a great ransom: moreover he bore in his hand the sceptre of the wreathed with a suppliant's wreath, and he besought the Achseans, but most of all the two sons of Atreus, who were their chiefs.
>
> "Sons of Atreus," he cried, "and all other Achseans, may the gods who dwell in Olympus grant you to sack the city of Priam, and to reach your homes in safety; but free my daughter, and accept a ransom for her, in reverence to Apollo, son of Jove." ([8] p. 21)

Achilles, by the will of his father Peleus, had studied medicine and pharmacy with the wise Chiron, who also counted Asclepius, whom we will deal with later in this discussion, among his disciples. Achilles as a student had the skills and potential to become a good doctor. A medicinal plant was even named after him, the Achillea, which, thanks to its active ingredients, carried out a precious pharmacological action. He taught his friend Patroclus some of the teachings he had learned. This is confirmed by Homer in book XI verses 844–848, in which Patroclus extracts the arrow from Eurypylus' thigh, washes the wound with warm water and applies a bitter root which calms the pain; the wound dries up and stops bleeding.

The Trojan War raged in the twelfth century BCE. A few centuries later, Homer describes the gods and demigods who mark the birth of the medical art. Podalirius and Machaon, sons of Asclepius, who, in turn, is the son of Apollo, are doctors in the Greek army; Hygeia and Panacea, both daughters of Asclepius, although from different mothers, establish themselves as goddesses of health and healing; Helen is skilled in the use of drugs; Chiron teaches Achilles, Theseus, Aeneas, Hercules and Diomedes. Cicero claims that Asclepius was a man. Man or god, he was certainly a character who left an indelible mark on the history of Western medicine and pharmacy. Tradition tells us that Mercury (Hermes), the messenger of the gods, received a staff from Apollo. When he arrived in Arcadia, two serpents devouring each other appeared before him, so he threw the staff between them and they made peace. From this legend was born the symbol of the caduceus, a sign of peace represented by a staff with two open wings and two coiled serpents looking at each other. For this reason, the caduceus became the symbol of heralds negotiating peace in ancient Greece. It was also considered a symbol of moral balance and exemplary conduct: the staff represents power; the two serpents, wisdom; the wings, diligence; and the helmet, the emblem of elevated thoughts. Asclepius, god of medicine, carried the caduceus; born from the union between Apollo and Coronis, he was a very good doctor and founded some temple-hospitals; he also created a medical school but, driven by ambition, began to resurrect the dead. This did not please Hades, god of the underworld, who complained to Jupiter; the latter, angry at such presumption, killed Asclepius with a thunderbolt. The caduceus used by Asclepius was represented by a single snake coiled around the staff, while the logo used by international medical associations preferred the one with two snakes. This was perhaps to represent the struggle between illness and healing and between life, death and rebirth—rebirth seen as a metaphysical or even psychological phenomenon in which renewal involves the abandonment of the old skin, composed of habits, prejudices and preconceptions. The snake crawled in the rooms of the temple-hospitals founded by Asclepius to lick the wounds; this symbol appears coiled around the staff of the god of medicine in all his representations. Wine was used as a medicine and solvent; blood was used as a restorative medicine in the hospitals of the time. Sea and thermal baths were practised; massages with oils, administration of herbs, nutrition and the cleansing of wounds were studied. The gods would visit the patient during sleep and reveal the therapy to them. The patient was placed in a condition of serenity, hope and hygiene, ready for recovery and healing.

1.9 Hippocrates

Hippocrates, born on the island of Kos, around 460 BCE and died in 370 BCE, was a practitioner and teacher of medicine in Athens. He was, according to the testimony of near contemporaries, such as Plato and Aristotle, the most famous doctor of his time and, according to a tradition that culminates in Galen, the founder of scientific medicine in Greece. Tradition has transmitted to us a corpus of around 70 works that are attributed to Hippocrates. He composed works from both a philosophical and a strictly medical point of view; the most famous is the Oath, probably influenced by the Pythagorean sect, which is reported below in its original version and in a modern adaptation.

> Oath of a Pharmacist
>
> The revised Oath was adopted by the AACP Board of Directors and the APhA Board of Trustees in November 2021. AACP member institutions should plan to use the revised Oath of a Pharmacist during the 2021–2022 academic year and with spring 2022 graduates.
>
> I promise to devote myself to a lifetime of service to others through the profession of pharmacy. In fulfilling this vow:
>
> I will consider the welfare of humanity and relief of suffering my primary concerns.
>
> I will promote inclusion, embrace diversity, and advocate for justice to advance health equity.
>
> I will apply my knowledge, experience, and skills to the best of my ability to assure optimal outcomes for all patients.
>
> I will respect and protect all personal and health information entrusted to me.
>
> I will accept the responsibility to improve my professional knowledge, expertise, and self-awareness.
>
> I will hold myself and my colleagues to the highest principles of our profession's moral, ethical and legal conduct.
>
> I will embrace and advocate changes that improve patient care.
>
> I will utilize my knowledge, skills, experiences, and values to prepare the next generation of pharmacists.
>
> I take these vows voluntarily with the full realization of the responsibility with which I am entrusted by the public. [13, 14]

Plato essentially says in *Phaedrus* that Hippocrates followed a method according to which it was not possible to cure a single disease and a single patient, "without knowing the nature of the whole". Central to this is the interpretation of the Platonic term "all" (*holon*). The "Hippocratic" treatises mark the birth of medical knowledge in written form, according to a process common in that period to other techniques (such as rhetoric, architecture and mathematics). The passage of the threshold of writing, accomplished by medicine in an impressive way both in the quality and quantity of works, had significant cultural consequences on the therapeutic art. First of all, it made the doctor a figure which belonged to the elite of cultured and prestigious intellectual professions. From closed and repetitive knowledge, transmitted through the generations from father to son and from master to disciple, the therapeutic art became an open and public technique, whose principles and methods became controllable and available for discussion and mutual refutation. Writing also allowed medicine to establish itself, from then on, as knowledge capable of combining the experiences of different professionals, therapeutic discoveries and dietary and pharmacological knowledge; in short, it inaugurated a medical tradition capable of development, conservation and innovation. The new medical knowledge was forced to emancipate itself from other methods of healing and beliefs. According to Hippocrates, diseases have a regular and predictable progression, often marked by attacks and remissions ("crises"). The cause of diseases is generally an imbalance between the body and the external environment (climatic conditions, excesses in lifestyle and especially incorrect nutrition), which gives rise to a further imbalance of the organic fluids within the body, the "humours", which can then be found in excessive or defective quantities, or be "raw" or too "cooked" (which is equivalent to not digested or retained in the organism for too long). The humours were reduced by the authors who interpreted the Hippocratic philosophy to four: blood, yellow and black bile and phlegm (catarrh). This identification of the four humours is evidently based on the observation of the main bodily excretions (faeces, urine, haemorrhages, catarrh and sweat), which (together with other manifestations of the patient) constitute for the Hippocratic physician the "signs" (or symptoms) from which they can diagnose pathological phenomena and, above all, predict the developments and outcomes of the disease. If the diagnosis and prognosis are based on the fluids exiting the body, the therapy will consist mainly of regulating the inputs and will be predominantly a dietary therapy (diet, however, concerns not only foods but the entire lifestyle, including, for example, sports exercises and baths). Pharmacological intervention is usually marginal and limited to vegetable infusions; bloodletting and surgery are practised, especially in the treatment of sprains and fractures. The scarcity of anatomical, physiopathological and pharmacological knowledge is compensated by an extraordinary attention paid to the person—the patient—rather than to the individual disease. Although it cannot be considered that Hippocratic medicine achieved significant successes regarding the main pathological conditions it had to deal with, it is certain that it was able to improve the living, hygienic and health conditions of its patients, from both a psychological and a dietetic point of view. In this sense, Hippocratic medicine constituted a reference model both methodologically and ethically until the nineteenth century.

1.10 The Romans: Dioscorides and Galen

There were many doctors who practised in Rome in the first decades of the Empire; among these, Dioscorides certainly stood out for his vast knowledge. He was also subsequently appreciated by Galen. Born in Asia Minor (40–90 CE), he studied in Greece and Alexandria and practised medicine as a soldier. After a lot of direct observation of plants in their native habitats and careful practical experience on the medicinal uses of herbs, as well as those derived from animals and minerals, Dioscorides wrote *De Materia Medica* in five books, "on the preparation, properties, and testing of drugs" (Preface, I), each chapter dealing with a single substance, its description, preparation and therapeutic properties. Dioscorides indicates in the Preface that, instead of presenting his *materia medica* ("the materials of medicine") in alphabetical order (which, he complains, "splits off genera and properties from what most resembles them"), "I shall endeavour to use a different arrangement and describe the classes according to the properties of the individual drugs" [15]. The scheme was to organize by category or class and then by the physiological effect of the drug on the body. This classification of drugs with similar pharmaceutical properties was too subtle to be readily comprehended, however, and was made even more obscure when, ironically, later copyists alphabetized the material, completely rearranging its original schema. *De Materia Medica* was the basis for pharmaceutical and herbal writing until the end of the sixteenth century. Although he was not a pharmacologist, he is considered to be the first to have written a treatise on pharmacology. The original treatise did not contain drawings, which were made by medieval illuminators during translations and copying. The University of Naples Federico Secondo together with the company Aboca has elaborated and republished the volume of Dioscorides integrating modern and contemporary knowledge. At this historical moment, another important figure stands out in Rome and his name will remain forever linked to the field of pharmacy that will be defined as Galenic. Today, we define an officinal Galenic preparation as a medicine prepared independently by the pharmacist in a pharmacy according to the pharmacopoeia of a member country of the European Union and intended to be dispensed directly to patients who use that pharmacy. Galen (born 129 CE in Pergamum, Turkey) was a Greek physician, writer and philosopher, whose influence dominated European medical theory from the Middle Ages to the seventeenth century. He also had a lasting impact on the Byzantine world and the Muslim Middle East. Galen was the son of a wealthy architect and initially trained as a philosopher. At 16, he shifted to studying medicine in Pergamum, Smyrna and Alexandria. After years of study, he returned to Pergamum in 157 CE to become the chief physician to a group of gladiators. In 162, he moved to Rome, where he gained fame through his public anatomy demonstrations, successful treatments of wealthy patients and debates. Galen's connections, including a friendship with his former philosophy teacher Eudemus, a student of Aristotle, helped further his career. In 166, he returned to Pergamum, possibly due to envy from colleagues or a plague in Rome. However, he was called back to Rome in 168–169 to accompany Emperors Lucius Verus and Marcus Aurelius on a military campaign. After Verus' death, Galen continued to serve as physician to subsequent emperors. His final works were written around 207 CE, and he is believed to have died in 216/217 at the age of 87.

1.11 The Birth of the Pharmacy as a Physical Place

Today, we all often go to the pharmacy for various reasons, but perhaps none of us ever think that until a few centuries ago there was no physical place where we could receive medicines or remedies that could help us heal even the most trivial diseases. This place is nowadays called a pharmacy, but, over time, it has had different names and places. In fact, we know that doctors, since ancient Rome, often produced medicines in the back of their surgeries with the help of technicians, as confirmed by Signore [16]. At this historical moment, the Romans started to see the patient and the necessity to care for them as a whole process; this is why we talk about *cura personalis*, as Bob Zebroski affirms in his book *A Brief History of Pharmacy: Humanity's Search for Wellness* [17]. The plants that were used were collected by external people, while resins, oils and fats were purchased. With Hellenism, this production increased more and more and the different operators became specialized, for example, the *herbarii* and *rhizomatoi*, who collected the plants and roots. Other terms used in this period were *pharmacopola*, *myrapola*, *medicamentarius, pigmentarius, aphotecarius* (storekeeper) and *aromatarius* (seller of aromatic spices). This is demonstrated by the sale deeds for pharmaceutical products found in this historical period. Some herbalists, having to import substances from distant countries, then transformed their businesses into *tabernae apothecariae*, which served as warehouses but sometimes also sold products to individual customers. In addition to the doctors themselves, there were also the *circulatores*, who brought their knowledge to remote places far from inhabited centres and always had with them the remedies for the most common illnesses. The *taberna seplasia* or *myrapolium* during the imperial period and throughout the Empire, from Rome to Constantinople to Ephesus, had a multifaceted activity as it sold perfumes, body-cleansing powders, soothing and scented ointments, prepackaged drugs or drugs to be prepared to a doctor's prescription to its customers-patients.

1.12 The Monks and the Islamic Golden Age

Ecclesiastical institutions, especially monasticism, became central forces in the birth of a new civilization during the period of the barbarian invasions. European monasticism, originating in the Middle East, is not exclusive to Christianity, but represents a universal spiritual quest. The hermetic life developed in Egypt, Palestine and Syria in the fourth century CE. Monasticism became a way to escape the worldliness of the church and preserve its spirituality. Initially characterized by a solitary and ascetic life, it was structured over time with the introduction of rules. The most famous was that of Saint Benedict of Nursia, who founded the monastery of Montecassino in the sixth century and wrote a rule that combined Roman practicality with Christian spirituality. This rule spread throughout Europe, with the help of Charlemagne, and profoundly influenced Western monasticism. Over the centuries, monasteries established themselves as centres of culture and spirituality, and many abbeys played an important role in the diffusion of culture and the transmission of texts related to the world of pharmacy and medicine.

In this context, the rise of Islam played a key role in advancing Arab medicine and pharmacy. The belief that God has provided a natural cure for every disease inspired the development of pharmacognosy. The Qur'an, as a moral guide for Muslims, shaped professional ethics, and the ritual of washing emphasized the importance of hygiene in preventative medicine. The knowledge of medicine spread throughout the Islamic Caliphate between the fall of the Roman Empire in the fifth century CE and the European Renaissance in the fifteenth century. However, the true flourishing of Arab medicine and pharmacy began in the ninth century, coinciding with the Golden Age of the Abbasid Caliphate (749–1258). With the establishment of the Abbasid Caliphate, major cultural and scientific activities shifted from Syria to Iraq. Baghdad, the newly founded city, became the empire's capital and a hub of culture and science. Other significant centres of learning included Damascus, Cairo and Cordoba and Granada in Spain, where institutions, schools, libraries and hospitals were built. These cities also saw the creation of the first pharmacies, attracting scholars and doctors from around the world to contribute to scientific progress. During this time, many books were translated into Arabic.

The most prominent figure of the translation movement was Hunayn ibn Ishaq al-Ibadi (809–873), who translated many works by Dioscorides, Hippocrates and Galen. The translation of Dioscorides' *De Materia Medica* in 1229 was especially important for medicine. This book was the first pharmacopeia enriched by Arab scholars, adding about 2000 substances. By the year 900, the Arab world had translated nearly all of the Greek scientific literature into Arabic. By comparison, European countries were less advanced, as they had access to poorly translated Arabic-Latin texts several years later.

The Islamic civilization deserves credit for having started to extract active ingredients with pharmacological action from herbs through alchemy, i.e. through chemical processes. Alchemy was born in the Hellenistic environment in Egypt in the first century CE and can be considered the progenitor of modern chemistry. Initially, the world of magic was linked to it and attempts were made to obtain compounds such as the elixir of long life, the drug that could give man eternal youth, and the remedy for all ills (panacea). The founder of Arab alchemy is probably Jabir ibn Hayyan, and several books are attributed to him in which reference is made to devices that allow the obtainment of chemical compounds through distillation, filtration and boiling. Essential oils began to be produced in this period. Pharmacy became an independent profession in the early ninth century, also thanks to Muslim scholars. The first hospitals with permanent pharmacies and apothecaries were established in Arab countries, marking the beginning of pharmacy as a distinct field from medicine, a distinction that began in the seventh century. Al-Biruni, a notable Arab scientist, emphasized that pharmacy aids medicine but is not a servant to it. Sabur (d. 869) wrote the first Arabic text on pharmacy, compiling formulas. The rise of pharmacy as an autonomous science was driven by factors such as increased drug demand, intellectual curiosity and the translation of medical texts. The opening of the first private pharmacy in Baghdad by Khalifa al-Mensur in 754 CE is often cited as a key moment in the independence of pharmacy from medicine. The first pharmacy in a hospital opened in Cairo in 873 CE.

1.13 The School of Salerno

It is said that a Greek pilgrim named Pontus stopped in the city of Salerno and found shelter for the night under the arches of the ancient Arce aqueduct. A storm broke out and another sick traveller took shelter in the same place, it was the Latin Salernus; he was wounded, and the Greek, at first suspicious, approached to observe closely the dressings that the Latin was providing to his wound. In the meantime, two other travellers had arrived, the Jew Elinus and the Arab Abdela. They also showed interest in the wound and in the end it was discovered that all four were involved in medicine. They then decided to create a partnership and start a school where their knowledge could be collected and disseminated. The *Schola Medica Salernitana* is considered the oldest medical school of modern civilization. Salerno's long medical tradition began during the Greco-Roman period in a Greek colony named Elea, where Parmenides decided to found a medical school. The fame of the school became increasingly important during the tenth century, and it was best known in the eleventh century. The school was at its apogee in the middle of the twelfth century, and Salerno provided a notable contribution to the formulation of a medical curriculum for medieval universities. The most famous work of the School of Salerno was the *Regimen Sanitatis Salernitanum*, a Latin poem of rational, dietetic and hygienic precepts, many of them still valid today. The school also produced a physician's reference book, with advice on how to treat a patient, a sort of code of conduct to help the physician to respect the patient and their relatives. The first science-based surgery appeared on the scene of the discredited medieval practice in Salerno, thanks to Roger of Salerno and his fellows. He wrote a book on surgery, called *Rogerina* or *Post Mundi Fabricam*, in which surgery from head to toe is described, with surprising originality. The important contribution to the School of Salerno made by women as practitioners is outlined, and among them, Trotula de Ruggiero was the most renowned. The period when the School of Salerno, universally recognized as the forerunner of the modern universities, became a government academy was when Frederick II reigned over the Kingdom of the Two Sicilies, as Emperor of the Holy Roman Empire.

1.14 Frederick II and the First Pharmacy in Europe

Two dates are very important in this historical journey that reconstructs the history of pharmacy: 1221 and 1241. The Middle Ages are often associated in the common sense with a dark and culturally insignificant period. In reality, the Middle Ages brought many advances in technology, economics and even politics. In the same era, the practice of pharmacy also changed, thanks to Emperor Frederick II of the Kingdom of the Two Sicilies. It was he who issued the Edict of Salerno, which was the law that prohibited doctors from also acting as pharmacists, when he noticed the rapid increase in the prices of medicines due to this practice; the edict, in fact, set the fixed price of some drugs. Frederick II, Emperor of the Holy Roman Empire and King of Sicily during the Middle Ages, noticed that the prices of medicines increased because doctors also did the work of pharmacists and created the drugs they prescribed. Frederick, known for his pursuit of knowledge and intellect, created the Edict or Constitution of Salerno in 1241. The edict decreed that the professions of physician and pharmacist were to be two separate and distinct professions. According to this decree, physicians could no longer practise pharmacy and the two professions could not be under one establishment. The edict soon became a model for regulating the practice of pharmacy throughout Europe. This is the first recognition of the social importance of pharmacy at a European level and the codification of professional behaviour on a regulatory level, so that it was clear that pharmacy, together with medicine, was an emanation of the state at the service of the citizen. It is no coincidence that Frederick II was nicknamed *stupor mundi* precisely because of his broad knowledge of the arts and sciences. The *Constitutiones*, in fact, embraced many spheres of law and contributed to the foundations for the birth of European law. A very significant step, for example, concerns a topic that is still much debated today, namely, economic violence against women within family law.

> Therefore, with this law of ours, which will be in force in all the individual parts of our kingdom, we establish that upon the death of the father, both sons and daughters, whether children or of greater or lesser age, are called to succeed to their parents without distinction of sex. [18]

The other key date is the birth of the first pharmacy in Europe, which is still open and can be visited by the public. The Officina Profumo-Farmaceutica di Santa Maria Novella has its roots in 1221. Founded as a convent of Dominican friars, it is today considered the oldest pharmacy in the world still in operation, although no longer a pharmacy but a perfumery. It all began 800 years ago, when the Dominican friars were granted the use of Santa Maria Inter Vineas (Saint Mary Among the Vines): It was a small church just outside the city walls, where they cultivated the botanical garden of aromatic herbs and plants to prepare medicines, ointments and balms. The Dominican friars of Santa Maria Novella became famous in 1334 for having healed the rich merchant Dardano Acciaioli: He came from one of the most powerful families in Florence, and as a sign of gratitude, he donated to the friars the magnificent chapel dedicated to San Niccolò, which is still located in the heart of the boutique-museum. Sometime later, in 1533, the Officina returned to be a protagonist in the history of European perfumery. It was in that year when the young Caterina de' Medici chose Renato Bianco, raised by the Dominican friars of Santa Maria Novella, to accompany her as her personal perfumer to the Court of France, where she was about to marry Henry II of Valois. Legend has it that *Acqua della Regina* was born on that occasion: a fragrance to recall the elegance and grace of Florence. The doors of the pharmacy officially opened to the general public in 1542, and it was formally recognized with the name of Officina Profumo-Farmaceutica by the Grand Duke of Tuscany in 1612, who also awarded it the title of the Foundry of His Royal Highness. Over the years, alongside traditional preparations, cosmetic and personal care products, such as balms, ointments, soaps and perfumes, became extremely popular. During the twentieth century, it became a boutique-museum, a much-visited tourist and cultural destination.

It was only in China, thanks to the reforms of the Song dynasty, that there was an Imperial Pharmacy, opened in 1076, which was a remarkable institution that played different political, social, economic and medical roles over the years of its existence. It was initially an economic institution designed to curb the power of plutocrats who were manipulating medicinal drug markets in their favour. A few decades later, the Imperial Pharmacy became a public-health-oriented institution focusing on selling ready-made prescriptions in addition to simples. Various records, including local gazetteers and local maps, indicate that the Imperial Pharmacy expanded about a century after it was established to include dozens of branches throughout the empire. Tallinn Town Hall Pharmacy is the oldest pharmacy in Europe that has continually operated on the same premises. It was first mentioned in town records in 1422. Frederick II's Edict of Salerno served as a stimulus throughout Europe for the opening of other pharmacies. Below is a list of the main pharmacies opening from the thirteenth century:

- Reavley Chemist is the oldest trading pharmacy in Burford, Oxfordshire. This building dates back to the year 1401.
- Pharmacie du Cerf was established in 1268 in Strasbourg, Alsace. It is the oldest pharmacy in France.
- Built in 1241, the "Löwen-Apotheke" in Trier is the oldest pharmacy in Germany and is protected as a historic monument.
- One of Austria's oldest chemist's shops, the "Apotheke zum Goldenen Biber", has been located in the Getreidegasse in Salzburg since 1608.
- Ferrein's Pharmacy was built in 1832 and renovated at the end of the nineteenth century; this elegant building featuring Neo-Renaissance and Baroque elements is renowned for hosting Moscow's oldest pharmacy.
- The Esteve Pharmacy is a medieval pharmacy and museum located in the town of Llívia, in the comarca of Cerdanya, Catalonia, Spain. It was founded at the beginning of the fifteenth century.
- Løveapoteket (lit. The Lion Pharmacy) was the first pharmacy in Copenhagen, Denmark. It opened in 1620 and operated until its closing in 1971, for a total of approximately 350 years.
- Swan Pharmacy or Svaneapoteket in Bergen, is the oldest pharmacy in Norway. It was established in 1595.
- Apoteket Lejonet (The Lion Pharmacy) was established in 1575 as Stockholm's first public pharmacy, originally named "Slottsapotek". Its symbol was a reclining lion, and it provided medicine for royalty and citizens during significant health crises, such as the plague.
- The Pharmacy Museum's pharmacy shop houses the oldest remaining pharmacy interior in Finland, dating back to 1858. The museum also includes workrooms for the self-sufficient pharmacy, i.e. the materials room, two laboratories and the herb room.

- Apteka Rektorska (Rector's Pharmacy) in Zamość is a historic pharmacy located in a Renaissance building. It is the oldest pharmacy still operating today in Zamość and the oldest pharmacy in Poland. It has been operating continuously since 1609.
- The Sibiu Pharmacy Museum is housed in a 1569 Gothic townhouse where the oldest pharmacy in Romania operated for over 150 years. The pharmacy was known as La Ursul Negru (The Black Bear).
- Dolan's Pharmacy on Columcille Street in Tullamore, Republic of Ireland, can be dated to 1795.
- Jacob Hooy was established in 1743, making it the oldest existing spice store in Amsterdam, the Netherlands, and possibly the oldest in the Western world.

The spread of printing and the discovery of the Americas allowed the widespread circulation of European recipe books throughout the world.

1.14.1 Pharmacy After Its Official Creation and Today

European pharmacies in the Renaissance were decorated with carved benches, with rich shelves containing medicines in elegant vases that reflected, with their grace, the artistic taste of this era in European countries. Towards the end of the sixteenth century, the first inspection visits to pharmacies were established and apothecaries gathered in special orders and corporations. The pharmacy saw its golden age in Europe at the end of the eighteenth century and the beginning of the nineteenth century. In the back room of the Köping pharmacy, thanks to Scheele, the famous Swedish chemist, malic, citric and gallic acids were prepared; uric acid was isolated; molybdenum, wolfram and chlorine were discovered; and oxygen was obtained independently of J. Priestley, an Anglo-American chemist and theologian. Friedrich Sertürner studied the effects of opium in the small apothecary of Einbeck in Hannover, using himself as an experimental subject, and isolated the first alkaloid, morphine (from Morpheus, the god of sleep). The affirmation of the independence of pharmacy from chemistry and medicine was the result of the contribution of the work of pharmacists such as the Germans Marggraf, who discovered the presence of sucrose in beetroot, and Klaproth, who discovered cerium, zirconium and titanium. In addition to these, the contribution of others, such as J.-B. Dumas, P. Pelletier, G. C. Poggendorff, J. Liebig, F. Mohr, J. G. Dragendorff, F. Selmi and R. Piria, was fundamental. Nowadays, the preparation of medicinal drugs occurs on an industrial level, but the scientific mission of the pharmaceutical profession has not changed. Today, especially after the COVID-19 pandemic, the role of the pharmacist is linked to a relationship with the community that makes this figure a point of reference that obviously does not replace the family doctor but is present within the community. Kesa Hatamoto's story is an example: She is a 102-year-old Japanese woman who is recognized by Guinness World Records as the world's oldest pharmacist. She started her career over 70 years ago at the recommendation of her father, who was looking forward to women's future success in society. Hatamoto works at a pharmacy from 10 a.m. to 6 p.m., 6 days a week, and expresses a desire to continue her career for the rest of her life. Before World War II, her relatives wanted her to marry after graduation, as women were expected to focus on the family. However, Hatamoto, influenced by her self-employed father, aspired to become a teacher or doctor. Her father encouraged her to become a pharmacist, as it would allow her to work long-term, even after marriage. She enrolled at Tokyo University of Pharmacy and Life Sciences, where the course was shortened due to the war. After graduating in 1942, she worked in a chemical plant lab before evacuating to Nagano due to air raids. After marrying at 25, she returned to Tokyo. Shortly after marriage, most of their assets were seized due to her husband's co-signed loan. At 30, she opened a pharmacy, following advice from an acquaintance of her husband. Reflecting on it, she described herself as naive but determined. Though she enjoyed her job, a relative once asked if she wanted to be a businesswoman, which Hatamoto found unusual. In April of last year, she was recognized as the world's oldest pharmacist at 101 years and 196 days. "Everyone is helping and being helped", Hatamoto said. "It would be great if (for each of us) there is something you could do your best at in the environment you are given" [19].

1.14.2 The Visit to the Noble College of Pharmaceutical and Chemical Sciences of Rome

Visiting the Church of San Lorenzo de' Speziali, located within the Roman Temple of Antoninus and Faustina, which directly overlooks the Roman Forum, feels like taking a journey back in time through various historical periods. Accompanied by two Noble Collegiate Members, Tito Piccioni and Giancarlo Signore, one walks through the church's nave, which houses paintings by Pietro da Cortona, Vanni, Domenichino, Alessandro Fortuna and other masters. Descending to the lower level, one can admire the private collection of Pharmaceutical Art and the History of Pharmacy, which includes albarelli (apothecary jars) from various eras, bronze mortars, laboratory instruments, antique glassware, medals from different periods, prints and old paintings. The library and archive preserve ancient manuscripts, old statutes, historic pharmacopoeias from different countries, texts from the sixteenth century and recently published works (Fig. 1.1).

The enlightened will of Pope Martin V granted the Collegiate Church of San Lorenzo—built within the ancient Roman temple—to the Guild of Roman Pharmacists on 8 March 1429 in recognition of its merits. (The original walls of the temple can still be seen inside the church.) Emperor Antoninus had the temple built in 142 BCE in honour of his wife Faustina. This donation fulfilled the Guild's wish to have a sacred space where they could gather in prayer and reflect on the Christian and social values of their art. In 1602, the Guild of Apothecaries decided to erect the

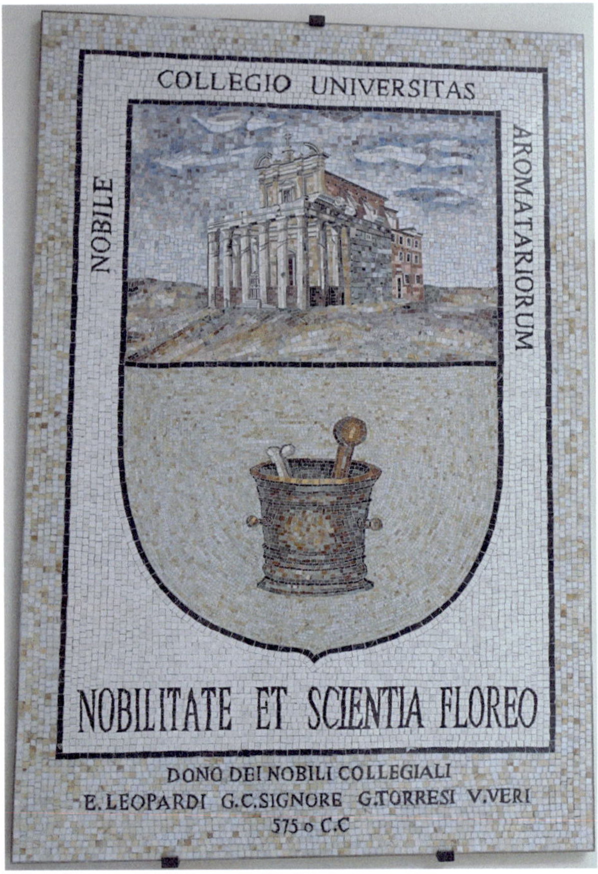
COLLEGIO UNIVERSITAS
NOBILE
AROMATARIORUM
NOBILITATE ET SCIENTIA FLOREO
DONO DEI NOBILI COLLEGIALI
E. LEOPARDI G.C.SIGNORE G.TORRESI V.VERI
575 o C.C

Fig. 1.1 Mosaic located in the private collection of Pharmaceutical Art and the History of Pharmacy, Rome. (Photographed by Horowitz Iris Oryah)

church still within the Roman temple, which, in all its splendour, remains a source of pride for the Imperial Forums, the city of Rome and Italian pharmacists. The church was named San Lorenzo de' Speziali in Campo Vaccino. Once the complex was completed, the Noble College of Apothecaries, by papal decree, was entrusted with institutional roles that today are the responsibility of the Ministry of Health, professional boards and universities.

These prerogatives ceased in 1871, with the annexation of Rome into the Italian State. The Noble Roman College of Pharmacists—the world's oldest institution of the pharmaceutical art—shifted its focus to academic, cultural and social functions. It is composed of 50 Noble Collegiate Members, who must meet criteria of professional and scientific merit and integrity and be practising pharmacists in Rome. These members promote research and studies in the history of pharmacy, pharmaceutical sciences and social health sciences, while also safeguarding the Church of San Lorenzo de' Speziali. Conferences, professional development courses and training on pharmaceutical subjects are still held there today.

1.14.3 Practice Time

1. Have you ever reflected on the figure of the pharmacist in your experience of study, research and work?
2. Do you think that non-European traditions related to medicine can teach us something even today?
3. Frazer's text describes the habits and traditions of different peoples around the world that deal with curing people and animals through various tools, even magic. Do you think this could be a text to recommend to your colleagues?
4. Do you think that the pharmacist's oath is a tradition to carry forward today?
5. Were you aware of the connection between Achilles and the practice of healing?
6. Have you ever visited or would you like to visit one of the ancient pharmacies mentioned in this chapter to better understand how this profession has been fundamental since it was emancipated from medicine?
7. Do you consider shamanism as one of the new therapeutic possibilities for neuropsychological disorders that are still difficult to treat, such as depression, anxiety, post-traumatic stress and chronic pain?

References

1. Laurent A, Laurent S. Le chamane et le médecin: Soigner, guérir. Paris: Odile Jacob; 2023.
2. Zink A, Samadelli M, Gostner P, Piombino-Mascali D. Possible evidence for care and treatment in the Tyrolean Iceman. Int J Paleopathol. 2019;25:110–7.
3. Deter-Wolf A, Robitaille B, Riday D, Burlot A, Jacobsen M. Chalcolithic tattooing: historical and experimental evaluation of the Tyrolean Iceman's body markings. Eur J Archaeol. 2024;27(3):267–88.
4. Frazer JG. The golden bough. London: Mcmillan; 1890.
5. Frazer JG. Totemism and exogamy: a treatise on certain early forms of superstition and society, vol. 4. London: Macmillan; 1910.
6. Frazer JG. Folk-lore in the old testament; studies in comparative religion legend and law. London: Macmillan; 1918.
7. Frazer JG. The magical origin of kings. London: Macmillan; 1920.
8. Butler S, editor. The Iliad of Homer. London: Longmans, Green, and Co; 1898.
9. Pugliarello R, Biolchi P, Cardini F. Medicina tradizionale cinese. In: Bellavite P, Conforti A, Lechi A, Menestrina F, Pomari S, editors. Le medicine complementari. Milan: UTET Periodici; 2000.
10. Pugliarello R, editor. Storia e teoria della medicina cinese. Milan: UTET Periodici; 2000.
11. Elferink JGR. The Inca healer: empirical medical knowledge and magic in pre-Columbian Peru. Rev Indias. 2015;75(264):323–50.
12. World Health Organization. Medicines. In: WHO health topics. Available from: https://www.who.int/health-topics/medicines#tab=tab_1.
13. McCollough Scholars Project. Hippocratic Oath (classical). University of Alabama. Available from: https://mccolloughscholars.as.ua.edu/hippocratic-oath-classic/.
14. U.S. Pharmacist's Oath. In: Pharmacist.com. Available from: https://www.pharmacist.com/About/Oath-of-a-Pharmacist.
15. Dioscorides P. De materia medica. ca. 50–70 CE.
16. Signore G. Storia della farmacia. Dalle origini al XXI secolo. Milan: Edra; 2013.

17. Zebroski B. A brief history of pharmacy: humanity's search for wellness. Abingdon: Routledge; 2015.
18. Mazzarese Fardella E. Appunti di storia del diritto medievale e moderno. Palermo: La Torre; 2003.
19. The Japan Times. At 102, world's oldest pharmacist celebrates her calling. 2025 Mar 6. Available from: https://www.japantimes.co.jp/news/2025/03/06/japan/oldest-pharmacist/.

Chapter 2
Care and Communication

2.1 Introduction

At a time when conflicts are spreading across the globe, just a few years after a global pandemic crisis, it has never been more important to reflect on communication, especially in the field of medical care. Through dialogue with others, we can learn, as Atlan argues, that treating the human being, rather than just the disease, can only be something extra, artificial in a certain sense, where caring for the person is like an epiphenomenon about which biology has nothing to say ([1] p. 20). The more scientific medicine is, the more it risks being depersonalized: this is what explains, above all, the fact that it arouses both fear and fascination. It is, therefore, essential to avoid the temptation to deify or demonize science. When faced with a feeling of helplessness concerning the injustices that occur around us every day, what we can do is try to take care of others.

The theoretical framework underlying this reflection integrates contributions from various disciplines. The concept of dialogical learning theorized by Ramón Flecha [2] is of fundamental importance; he, in turn, draws inspiration from thinkers, such as Lev Vygotsky [3], Paolo Freire [4], Jerome Bruner [5] and Jürgen Habermas [6]. According to Vygotsky [3], cognitive development is socially mediated and occurs through linguistic interaction: The zone of proximal development[1] is activated thanks to dialogue between peers and the support of more expert figures. Similarly, Bruner [5] emphasized the role of culture and narrative in the construction of the mind: thought develops through stories and shared language. Freire, in his *Pedagogy of the Oppressed* [4], proposes an emancipatory vision of education based on dialogism, bottom-up participation, awareness-raising and the critical capacity of individuals and communities. Habermas [6] enriches the conceptual framework by introducing the concept of communicative action: authentic

[1] This theme will be further developed in Chap. 3.

S. Leoncini, *The Relationship between Pharmacists and Patients*, New Paradigms in Healthcare, https://doi.org/10.1007/978-3-032-21249-8_2

communication, based on the search for consensus through valid arguments, becomes an instrument of social transformation. Language, therefore, is not only a vehicle of meaning but an instrument of action, and speaking, discussing and exchanging ideas are performative acts that modify reality [7]. Added to these references are the contributions of George Mead [8], according to whom the self is constructed through interaction with others, and of Hans-Georg Gadamer [9], who highlighted the importance of dialogical hermeneutics in understanding texts and the world.

The idea of care has woven itself through human thought like a golden thread, appearing in mythology, religion, philosophy, psychology and everyday practice. Rather than forming a single, rigid doctrine, care represents a constellation of related concepts, united by common concerns, recurring motifs and foundational stories that have shaped moral imagination across cultures and eras. The English word *care* carries a rich etymological history, tracing back to the Middle High German *kar* and the Common Teutonic *caru*, which conveyed trouble or grief, a sense of burdened concern. This ancestral meaning lingers, reminding us that true care always involves vulnerability. Over time, the term has branched into four interconnected senses: anxiety or sorrow, the weight of worry; investment or commitment, dedication to people; causes or ideals, responsible action, the practical work of "taking care" of tasks; and tender devotion, nurturing others' growth. These meanings sometimes pull in different directions. Is care a duty or an emotional bond, a professional service or a personal connection? Such tensions reveal care's dialectical nature; it can liberate or constrain, empower or smother, mend or damage. Many traditions, from ancient myths to modern psychology, position care as essential to being human. It is the soil in which moral awareness grows, fostering responsiveness to others and a sense of obligation. Yet, despite its significance, care has often been marginalized in formal ethical theories, which tend to prioritize abstract rules over relational wisdom.

Care has appeared in various ethical frameworks historically without being systematized:

Evolutionary ethics—caregiving as key to human survival
Virtue ethics—care as a moral character trait
Growth-centred ethics—such as Mayeroff's vision of nurturing potential [10]
Relational ethics—duties arising from interdependence
Duty ethics—adapted to caregiving contexts

Yet care resists reduction to mere "caregiving". The ancient *Myth of Care* suggests something deeper: that care is woven into human nature, shaping psychology, culture and society. It proposes that being well cared for is a prerequisite for flourishing a counternarrative to purely individualistic or transactional views of morality.

Though long overshadowed by impersonal ethical systems, care is now reclaiming attention, particularly in healthcare ethics. This revival reflects its dual role: care is both emotional and practical, demanding sensitivity to its rhythms, limits and risks. It also operates across generations, influencing identity and moral development throughout life. At its heart, the ethics of care rests on a vision of humanity as fundamentally relational, capable of giving and receiving care, and morally obligated to do so with wisdom and compassion. It challenges us to rethink responsibility, not as abstract duty but as active, attentive engagement with the world and one another.

In the end, care is more than a feeling or a task. It is a way of being in the world, one that calls individuals and institutions alike to foster connection, nurture growth and honour our shared vulnerability.

2.2 The Concept of Care Through Different Perspectives

According to Hyginus' anthropogony, expressed in the Roman *Myth of Cura*, Cura crosses a river and, on the other side, bends down to the earth to pick up a clump of clay. From that clay, she shapes the being that will become man. Jove comes along and Cura asks him to give life to the artefact. Jove complies and gives the gift of spirit to the shape formed by Cura, but a quarrel erupts over the name of the new creation. Should it be named after Cura or after the male celestial god? At this stage, Tellus, the god of earth, intervenes and claims Cura's creation, arguing that he provided the material from which it was formed. Saturn, the god of time, settles the matter through an act of naming and by dividing and temporalizing the possession of the various parts that comprise man: Jove is offered man's soul and Tellus his body after man's death, while Cura will possess the creation in its lifetime since she made it. Saturn names the new being "homo" because it was originally shaped out of humus. Thus, human life as a composite assembly of spiritual (Jove) and material elements (Tellus) is held together by Cura's temporal care.

The name Cura is derived from the verb *curo*. The Oxford Latin Dictionary defines the verb thus:

1. To watch over, look after, care for.
2. To tend to, to do what is necessary to.
3. To administer remedies, to treat (a sick person, wound, disease,
4. etc.).
5. To have charge of, (absol.) to be in command.
6. To devote oneself to, to cultivate (a person).
7. To undertake, to see to (a task or a responsibility).
8. To regard with anxiety or interest, worry or care about, heed [11].

I decided to evoke the Roman *Myth of Cura* to unpack theoretical understandings of care [12]. In this myth, known from the writings of the first-century mythographer Hyginus, humanity is created from clay by a personification of care. It has proven useful to thinkers as diverse as Martin Heidegger [13], Arthur Kleinman [14] and Julia Kristeva [15]. While utilization by Heidegger [13] challenges the myth of self-sufficiency and individual atomization that has shaped much of modern Western philosophy, both Kleinman [14] and Kristeva [15] explore the tension between universalized knowledge and the singularity of individual patients and intimate care.

Concepts such as justice, liberty and love have taken precedence for much of Western philosophy, while care remained a marginal concern until many scholars in the 1980s introduced a "care perspective" into moral discourse, particularly in bioethics. Yet, this modern framing often neglects earlier traditions where care, though not explicitly named, played a vital and complex role. In ancient Roman thought, the Latin *cura* carried two contrasting meanings: it could signify oppressive anxiety or devoted, meticulous attention [16]. Virgil portrayed the Curae as tormenting spirits at the gates of the underworld, while Seneca celebrated *cura* as a divine attribute, a force that elevates humanity by guiding it towards virtue [17]. This duality, care as both burden and moral excellence, is vividly captured in Hyginus' *Fabulae*, where a myth presents human existence as fundamentally shaped by Cura. Unlike theories rooted in competition or social contracts, this narrative suggests that human identity and community arise from shared fragility and the necessity of mutual attentiveness. Here, care is not just an individual duty but the very foundation of societal cohesion, the "binding thread" that sustains collective life. The myth also implies a radical rethinking of power: Humans are named not after gods but after humus (earth), emphasizing groundedness and interdependence. Those who receive care are not merely passive; being nurtured from birth enables them, in turn, to nurture others, a perspective supported by developmental psychology.

Beyond mythology, the ancient concept of *cura animarum* (care of souls) offers another precursor to modern care ethics. This practice across religious and philosophical traditions involved holistic healing—tending to physical, emotional and spiritual suffering through compassion, guidance and reconciliation. The "soul" here referred not just to religious essence but to the entirety of a person's inner life and moral being. Socrates famously prioritized the soul's welfare over material wealth, while early Christian theologians, such as Gregory the Great, framed spiritual leaders as "healers of the soul", tasked with mending psychological and ethical wounds. This form of care was deeply relational, requiring empathetic engagement with suffering. Biblical texts, such as Psalm 142's lament, "No one cares for my soul", highlight the anguish of neglect, while the New Testament contrasts life's oppressive burdens with divine solace. These traditions recognized that true care must address not only tangible needs but also the profound, often unspoken dimensions of human existence.

According to the theory of physicist Jean-Émile Charon (1920–1998), the characteristics of living beings, including the spiritual characteristics of humans, are due to the electrons that constitute them [18], whose mass for a 70 kg man can be calculated at 21 grams [19]. This value corresponds to the loss of mass observed by Duncan MacDougall (1866–1920), an American physician who in 1901 attempted to measure the "weight of the soul" [19], assuming that it leaves the human body at death. This singular coincidence served as input for the author's research hypothesis on life after death, which justifies experiences such as déjà vu, reincarnation and synchronistic events. This inspired Alejandro Iñarritu, who in the film of the same name ("21 grams"), starring a magnificent performance by Sean Penn, makes us reflect on the weight of the soul.[2]

Going back to the concept of care, centuries after, Johann Wolfgang von Goethe revived the *Myth of Care* in *Faust* [20]. Influenced by Johann Gottfried Herder's *Das Kind der Sorge* (*The Child of Care*) ([21] pp. 743–4), Goethe's main character seeks limitless knowledge, rejecting care's constraints in a pact with Mephistopheles. Yet, Faust's pursuit of power leads to moral decay, culminating in a confrontation with Sorge (care), who blinds him, a moment of reckoning that paradoxically grants him clarity. In his final moments, Faust shifts from selfish ambition to envisioning a just society, suggesting that care, though painful, holds redemptive power. Goethe's tale reframes care as not just personal compassion but a collective ethical imperative. Søren Kierkegaard further transformed care into an existential principle. Rejecting detached rationality, he argued that authentic living demands passionate engagement, a "concerned thinker" who confronts life's uncertainties with moral urgency [22]. For him, care was the essence of selfhood: the drive to shape one's existence through meaningful choices. He also explored care's paradox, its capacity to weigh heavily yet also inspire spiritual growth, communal solidarity and even divine connection. Heidegger later placed Sorge (care) at the heart of human existence [13]. Expanding on Kierkegaard, he defined care as the core of Dasein ("being-in-the-world"), encompassing both practical engagement (*Besorgen*) and ethical concern for others (*Fürsorge*). He cautioned against inauthentic care, either domineering interference or passive indifference. True care, he argued, requires confronting life's finitude and ambiguity, echoing the ancient *Myth of Care*.

[2] In Inarritu's movie, Jack Jordan is a former prisoner who became a fundamentalist Christian after his final stint. His family life is made difficult by his insistence on faith, which often veers into fanaticism, while his chances of finding work are compromised by his criminal record. Cristina is a former cocaine addict and alcoholic who now lives a quiet life with her husband and two daughters. Paul Rivers is a mathematician with serious heart problems, awaiting a donor for a delicate heart operation; due to his illness, he finds himself living with his ex-wife Mary, again. Despite not wanting children with him when they were married, Mary now insists on having a child with him through artificial insemination, fearing Paul's death. The pivotal event around which the entire story revolves is the car accident in which Jack Jordan hits Cristina's husband and daughters, who die due to the hit-and-run. The heart of Cristina's husband, Michael, is implanted in Paul Rivers, who, now healed, can finally return to his life, although he simultaneously develops an obsessive desire to know who the donor is to whom he owes his life. He, thus, comes upon Cristina, who, to escape the pain of losing her husband and daughters, has fallen back into a spiral of drug and alcohol addiction. Paul manages to get to know her and establish a relationship with her, which initially seemed compromised by the tragic circumstances that had bound them. Meanwhile, Paul is experiencing symptoms of rejection of the transplanted heart and, unwilling to undergo another operation with an uncertain outcome, obtains a gun to commit suicide. He and Cristina, wanting to avenge the death of Cristina's family, decide to kill Jack Jordan, who, in the meantime, had turned himself in—driven by remorse—and has already served his sentence. The two track him down to a squalid hotel where he has chosen to live as a semi-recluse, far from his family. Paul will try to kill him but, in the end, will choose to spare him, allowing him to continue a life that Jack himself, torn by guilt, would have wanted to end. This will lead to the final meeting between the three characters and the dramatic conclusion of the story.

Philosopher Milton Mayeroff presents a deeply personalist vision of care that transcends traditional ethical frameworks in his seminal work *On Caring* [10]. Moving beyond abstract principles, he anchors care in the concrete reality of human relationships, where helping another "grow", whether a person, idea or community, becomes the fundamental moral act. He conceptualizes care as an active, reciprocal process of fostering another's autonomous development. A teacher caring for a student, for instance, means supporting the student's unique path of becoming while resisting the temptation to impose predetermined outcomes. This relationship proves mutually transformative, as we care for others, we ourselves grow in understanding and capability. The cared-for person's flourishing becomes integral to the caregiver's own sense of purpose and fulfilment.

Mayeroff makes a crucial distinction between authentic care and goal-oriented interventions. Where a doctor might focus narrowly on curing symptoms, true care requires being fully present to the patient's experience. He warns against reducing relationships to measurable results, emphasizing instead care as a way of being characterized by essential qualities of care: devotion, trust, respect for the other's autonomy, patience, empathic knowledge and moral courage. Effective caring, Mayeroff observes, follows a natural rhythm of engagement and withdrawal. Overbearing attention often signals the caregiver's anxiety rather than a genuine concern for the other's development. True care knows when to step back, allowing space for independent growth while remaining available when needed. Mayeroff proposes care as the basis for an "ethics of response"—obligations emerging organically from relationships rather than abstract rules. When we commit deeply to caring, it naturally organizes our values and gives coherence to our lives. This perspective anticipates contemporary care ethics by prioritizing relational context over universal principles, valuing emotional engagement as morally significant and recognizing interdependence as fundamental to human flourishing. Ultimately, he positions care at the existential centre of human life. Our sense of meaning arises from both being needed by others and receiving care ourselves. His vision echoes ancient understandings of care while offering fresh insights for modern applications in education, therapy and healthcare—reminding us that in helping others grow, we ourselves become more fully human. His work endures as a profound meditation on how caring relationships shape our moral development, our understanding of responsibility and our very sense of purpose in the world.

2.3 Listen to the Patient: The Role of Empathy

> As is so often the case in neurology, reports of quirky and bizarre cases were among the early clues to the brain basis of empathy. A 1975 report, for instance, reviewed several cases in which patients with certain lesions in the right area of the frontal lobes had a curious deficit: they were unable to understand the emotional message in people's tone of voice, though they were perfectly able to understand their words. A sarcastic "Thanks," a grateful "Thanks," and an angry "Thanks" all had the same neutral meaning for them. By contrast, a 1979 report spoke of patients with injuries in other parts of the right hemisphere who had

> a very different gap in their emotional perception. These patients were unable to express their own emotions through their tone of voice or by gesture. They knew what they felt, but they simply could not convey it. All these cortical brain regions, the various authors noted, had strong connections to the limbic system. These studies were reviewed as background to a seminal paper by Leslie Brothers, a psychiatrist at the California Institute of Technology, on the biology of empathy. Reviewing both neurological findings and comparative studies with animals, Brothers points to the amygdala and its connections to the association area of the visual cortex as part of the key brain circuitry underlying empathy. [...] ([23] p. 78)

Research conducted by psychologist Robert Levenson at the University of California, Berkeley, provides evidence for a physiological foundation of empathy in humans [24]. Levenson employed a straightforward methodology in his studies of married couples engaged in emotionally charged discussions, such as disagreements over parenting strategies or financial decisions. The interactions were recorded on video, while physiological data, such as heart rate and skin conductance, were collected simultaneously. Subsequently, each partner viewed the recording twice: firstly, to narrate their own emotional experiences during the conversation, and then to interpret the emotional state of their spouse at each moment. Findings revealed that the highest levels of empathic accuracy were observed in individuals whose physiological responses closely mirrored those of their partner. A rise in one partner's skin conductance, for example, was matched by a similar increase in the other, and decreases in heart rate were similarly mirrored. This physiological synchronization appeared to be a critical marker of empathy. Conversely, individuals whose bodily responses merely replicated their own original patterns during the interaction demonstrated poor insight into their partner's emotional state. Thus, empathy was present only when there was a physiological resonance with the other person. These results imply that intense emotional arousal, such as during episodes of anger, may inhibit empathic processes. Empathy, it seems, necessitates a state of emotional composure and openness, allowing for the accurate reception and internal simulation of another's subtle affective cues.

Both Daniel Goleman [23] and Antonio Damasio [25] offer perspectives that transcend the Cartesian view. Specifically, the Portuguese scholar Damasio develops the theory of somatic markers, according to which emotions emit bodily signals that alert us to faster decision-making. This view distinguishes between emotions (automatic bodily responses) and feelings (emotional awareness). These two scholars offer concepts of empathy that, while converging on certain aspects, differ in their underlying theoretical approach. Damasio, from a neurobiological perspective, interprets empathy as a phenomenon rooted in bodily and emotional processes, closely linked to the mechanisms of homeostasis and the interaction between feeling and consciousness. Goleman, on the other hand, places empathy within emotional intelligence, emphasizing the social and relational dimension of emotional understanding of others, with a greater focus on interpersonal skills and self-reflection. While Damasio identifies empathy as an expression of emotional physiology, Goleman considers it an essential component of social competence, functional to the effective management of relationships. For Damasio, consciousness is divided into three levels: proto-consciousness (proto-self), core consciousness (core self) and autobiographical consciousness (autobiographical self). Proto-consciousness is a coherent set of neural configurations that create, moment by moment, maps of the state of the organism's physical structure in its many dimensions. It is a constantly updated set of neural configurations that regulates the basic functions for our survival. When an object changes the neural maps of proto-consciousness, a first form of conscious activity begins. Core consciousness, on the other hand, comes into play when neural structures "represent", nonverbally or through images, something of the external world, something of the changes in our organism, i.e. those changes caused by the perception of the object, a perception that makes the image of the object more vivid, an object that is contextualized in space and time. The object can be perceived (external) or recalled (internal). Core consciousness, thus, enters an experiential continuum both through the continuous flow of perceptions of the objects around us and when objects are evoked or recalled from memory. The flow of perceptions, in which we are immersed, modifies our proto-consciousness, objects modify its state and the flow of consciousness is modulated by many objects simultaneously. Proto-consciousness is not a conscious state of consciousness. Core consciousness is the first conscious level of consciousness; it corresponds to "being able to feel emotion". Nuclear consciousness is a brain configuration that is modified by the effects produced by an object that alters the perception of bodily states. It does not involve language, and since we are always immersed in the presence of objects, which trigger conscious experience, this is how our continuous perception of time emerges, a perception that prolongs consciousness over time. Nuclear consciousness requires proto-consciousness as a precondition. Core consciousness creates the "sense" of a certain time and place. It is a phenomenon independent of memory, language, reason or our actions. In other words, core consciousness is the effect of the organism's encounter with an object. It corresponds to the changes the organism undergoes upon encountering the object. Unlike proto-consciousness, core consciousness can represent any object. Proto-consciousness, i.e. the "(cerebral) representation of the organism", is a prototype of core consciousness; it is its biological version, the biological version of the sense of self. For Damasio, feelings are formed thanks to core consciousness, i.e. thanks to the ability to feel emotions. In core consciousness, the organism is projected at the brain level as a unit within structures that continuously receive signals from the internal states of the body. It is "instantaneous" (here and now) object consciousness, a-conceptual or non-reflective. It is associated with a pre-reflective sense of subjectivity derived from bodily representation. It guarantees a sense of self at a given moment, in the present. It is a first-level mapping. The projection of the object is configured in a brain map that involves the sensory and motor areas stimulated by the organism's encounter with the object. It is the sensation of the present, of what is happening in the moment, and consists of the production of mental "images" that underlie our raw experience: a wooden table, a coloured surface, a noise, a bodily sensation of well-being. These images are neural patterns represented as a whole by the organism. Core consciousness characterizes not only humans but also many non-human animals. Organism and object, as neural configurations, are projected into first-level maps. These neural configurations can transform into images. The sensorimotor maps related to the object produce modifications in the maps related to the organism. The sensorimotor maps related to the object modify the maps related to our organism (which is modified following interaction with the object). These modifications can, in turn, be represented in second-level maps that summarize the organism-object interaction. The neural configurations we encounter in second-level maps are temporary and can convert into images, as has already happened with the configurations in first-level maps. Therefore, consciousness would be the effect of this process of constructing mental images generated by the organism-object relationship. The maps of the organism, both first- and second-level, are linked to the body. The relationship between organism and object is described by mental images that correspond to feelings. The sensation that emerges from the (secondary) representation of proto-consciousness (non-conscious) when modified by its interaction with the object, thus, becomes the basis of core consciousness. The descriptions and narratives we make about our interactions with the object are the basis on which autobiographical consciousness is formed. This consciousness represents the "feeling we have of knowing", a sensation that allows us to know that we exist as subjects, in the act of knowing, as subjects of a narrated story. Autobiographical consciousness is also called "extended consciousness" and represents the ability to keep track of our history, to have a coherent perception of our personal events. It is nourished by memories from autobiographical memory concerning past experiences and predictions for the future; it is based on those recordings of the experiences of core consciousness that are activated and transformed into images. It should be emphasized that damage to core consciousness radically compromises the entire functioning of autobiographical consciousness, while impairment of the latter does not affect the functioning of core consciousness. Autobiographical consciousness is an extension, an expansion of core consciousness, on which it continues to depend; thanks to this extension, core consciousness is now projected into the past and the future, thanks to autobiographical narration. Autobiographical consciousness is the effect of the preservation of memories of numerous examples of a class of objects specific to our biography. Each autobiographical memory becomes an object for the brain, which activates core consciousness. It keeps the numerous collected images active, for a long time and simultaneously, and this structures what Damasio calls the autobiographical self [25].

Erica Francesca Poli tells about one of the first cases she worked on at the beginning of her career in her book *Healing Emotions* [26]. The patient was a 17-year-old transplant recipient, whom the author calls Cristina (using a pseudonym), who had rejected her kidney. The girl, already suffering from severe kidney failure and depression after the onset of rejection, initially refused to take any medication or see a psychologist. Her encounter with Dr. Poli changed everything, and the empathy the doctor developed with the patient allowed Poli to delve into the origins of the trauma that had led the girl to abandon her treatment. It was discovered that the rejected kidney had been donated by her mother, with whom the girl had a difficult relationship, described as overly normative and cold. Her actions were, therefore, not understood or metabolized by her daughter when the doctors decided to operate. Dr. Poli, using eye movement desensitization and reprocessing methodology, which is particularly suited to treating trauma, was able to rework with Cristina the events that led her to unconsciously somatize the pain related to those events. Cristina then underwent another transplant with another donor, and this time the operation was successful.

Reading Cristina's story, marked by pain, hope and disillusionment, elicits a profound emotional resonance in the reader. This phenomenon can be attributed to the activation of mirror neurons, a neural mechanism that enables us to internally simulate the emotions and experiences of others, even in the absence of direct personal experience. Through this system, the boundaries between self and others momentarily blur, allowing us to perceive Cristina's fear and resilience as if they were partially our own. When Dr. Poli recounts the episode of transplant rejection, a strong empathetic response is triggered. This response is facilitated by the brain's inherent capacity to understand and reflect the emotional states of others. Mirror neurons, in this context, serve as crucial neurobiological substrates underpinning empathy and intersubjective connection.

Mirror neurons were first discovered in 1992 by an Italian research team from Parma University guided by Giacomo Rizzolatti [27]. These neurons play a crucial role in our brain, allowing us to imitate actions, understand the mental states of others and form social bonds. Mirror neurons are a special type of neurons that activate when we both perform an action and observe someone else perform the same action. In other words, these neurons allow us to imitate what we see and understand the actions of others. This mechanism helps us learn through observation and develop a deeper understanding of the emotional states of others. One of the most fascinating aspects of mirror neurons is their role in empathy. When we see someone suffer or experience joy, our mirror neurons activate, allowing us to empathize and share the other's emotions. This is a key element in forming social bonds and helping individuals connect on a deeper level. Furthermore, mirror neurons play an important role in understanding the intentions of others. They allow us to "read" the mental states of others, understanding their motivations and desires. This ability is crucial for navigating the complex world of social interactions. Mirror neuron research has important implications for understanding disorders related to empathy and imitation. As an example, their inability to function properly has been associated with autism spectrum disorders, in which empathy and imitation can be limited. A better understanding of how these neurons function could lead to new therapeutic approaches for these conditions. The discovery of mirror neurons has led to an explosion of research in social neuroscience. Scientists continue to explore the diverse functions of these neurons and their impact on understanding human behaviour. Neuroimaging techniques, such as functional magnetic resonance imaging, have made it possible to observe the activation of mirror neurons in the human brain in real time, opening up new avenues for study. In conclusion, mirror neurons play a fundamental role in the formation of social bonds and the acquisition of knowledge through observation. Research continues on this topic, promising to reveal further secrets about the complex yet fascinating nature of the human brain. Mirror neurons are fundamental to our ability to feel and understand the emotions of others, and they are the neurological basis of empathy and emotional connection. But how long does an emotion last?

Emotions are neurohormones, chains of amino acids that travel through the brain and body carrying messages. Produced primarily in the hypothalamus, these chemicals affect literally every living cell in our body and are part of our primary regulatory function. Each burst of these chemicals, from the moment they are fully broken down and absorbed, lasts 5–7 s. Therefore, if we miss the opportunity of these 6 s, we lose the wisdom and energy that feelings offer; furthermore, if we feel something for more than 6 s, we are, on some level, choosing to recreate and replenish those feelings [28].

Rollo May, a pioneering voice in humanistic psychology, played a crucial role in bringing existentialist thought, particularly Heidegger's concept of care (Sorge), into the realm of psychological and moral discourse. His work bridged abstract philosophy and the lived struggles of the individual, making existential themes accessible to American audiences. In *Love and Will* [29], written during the 1960s, May identified a widespread psychological crisis marked by detachment, indifference, and disillusionment, what he called the "defining afflictions of our time" ([29] p. 306). He saw the era's youth rebellions not merely as political acts but as reactions to a deeper existential void, a gnawing sense that nothing truly mattered. For May, this pervasive apathy posed a dire threat to human vitality, and its cure lay in care: the deeply held belief that something, or someone, matters. May framed care not as a fleeting emotion but as an essential psychological stance, an active "rejection of meaninglessness" and a defiant affirmation of one's own existence. Influenced by Heidegger and the ancient *Myth of Care*, he asserted that care is fundamental to human identity, as care is the substructure of what it means to exist. To abandon care, he warned, is to surrender one's very being; thus, reclaiming care becomes a path back to genuine selfhood and ethical commitment. May saw care as the seed of conscience, its roots, he argued, stretch back to infancy: A child's survival hinges on being nurtured, and their early experiences of suffering become the foundation for later empathy. Ultimately, he positioned care as the psychological basis of ethics, an innate ability to look beyond oneself and act for the good of others. By linking care to conscience and empathy, May grounded ethics in human relationality rather than abstract rules. His legacy endures in psychology and beyond, reminding us that care is not passive but a courageous stance, one that resists despair and reaffirms our shared humanity. Regarding dialogue and listening, we can argue that within the perspective of education as a dialogical, democratic and transformative practice, speech is an instrument of freedom. As Freire stated [4], authentic speech, which transforms the world, implies an encounter. This is the context in which the communicative methodology adopted to implement these educational actions is based, which actively involves users throughout the entire research process, both as contributors to a richer understanding of their life-worlds and in the formulation of more effective educational policy solutions based on the most reliable scientific evidence available. This co-construction process is based on the dialogical relationship between the researcher and the social actors, or rather, the subjects involved in the research. The former provide knowledge and stimuli from the scientific community, while the latter provide insights based on the construction of meaning in relation to everyday life and the research topics, contributing to enriching the debate, for example, by examining doubts and challenges not initially contemplated and proposing alternative solutions. A significant metaphor is offered by Ahmed, a young man of Tunisian origin welcomed in Vittoria. During a Dialogic Literary Gathering (DLG) dedicated to the Odyssey, he compared Ulysses' journey to his own migration, sparking intense, empathetic discussion with all his classmates. In all the contexts monitored, the DLG methodology fostered the construction of a plural "we", as Flecha argues [2], in which cultural diversity became a shared resource, rather than a reason for exclusion.

2.4 Assertive, Passive and Aggressive Communication

The axioms of human communication formulated by the Palo Alto School, particularly by Paul Watzlawick and his collaborators [30], represent a fundamental theoretical framework for understanding the dynamics of communicative processes. They describe the inevitable and complex nature of interpersonal communication, highlighting how every exchange between individuals involves not only the transmission of information but also the construction and negotiation of relationships. The first axiom states that one cannot communicate: Every behaviour, including silence or apparent inactivity, has communicative value because it is interpreted by others. Communication is, therefore, not limited to spoken language but is inherent in every human act within a relational context. The second axiom establishes that every communication comprises both a content aspect and a relational aspect. Beyond the literal meaning of words, each communicative act defines the type of relationship connecting the participants, through tone, attitude, posture and other signals that qualify the interaction. The third axiom emphasizes that the nature of a relationship depends on the punctuation of the communication sequences. This means that each interlocutor tends to organize exchanges according to their own interpretation of cause and effect, attributing an order to events that often differs from that of other participants. Such discrepancies in "punctuation" may lead to misunderstandings and conflict. The fourth axiom highlights the dual modality of communication, which can be analogical and digital. Digital communication corresponds to verbal language, codified and structured, while analogical communication encompasses all nonverbal signs, such as gestures, facial expressions and intonation, that convey implicit meanings, emotions and relational nuances. Finally, the fifth axiom distinguishes between symmetrical and complementary interactions. Symmetrical interactions occur when interlocutors perceive themselves as being on an equal footing, whereas complementary interactions arise when the relationship is defined by differing roles, characterized by a "high" and "low" position that complement each other. In conclusion, these axioms show that human communication is an inevitable, continuous and multilayered process in which the relational and informational dimensions are inseparable. Understanding these principles allows for a deeper analysis of interpersonal dynamics and a more conscious interpretation of communicative behaviour [29]. Communication between pharmacist and patient is a fundamental element in ensuring a service that is effective, safe and person-centred. The manner in which the pharmacist interacts with individuals entering the pharmacy affects not only their understanding of prescribed therapies and adherence to treatment regimens but also their trust in and overall satisfaction with the healthcare experience.

Different communication styles may emerge within these interactions:

Assertive communication: this is the most effective and professionally appropriate approach. It enables the pharmacist to provide information, guidance and recommendations in a clear and respectful manner while actively listening to the patient and addressing their specific needs.

Passive communication: this occurs when the pharmacist avoids expressing necessary instructions clearly or refrains from intervening in the presence of a problem, thereby creating the risk of confusion and failing to provide adequate support.

Aggressive communication: characterized by harsh tones, imposing attitudes or a lack of active listening, this style may undermine the relationship of trust and negatively affect the patient's well-being. Adopting an assertive, patient-centred communication style is, therefore, essential to transform every interaction in the pharmacy into a genuine opportunity for support and care.

Assertiveness is the ability to clearly and effectively express one's emotions and opinions without overwhelming the other person. The goal is, therefore, identical to that of the aggressive and manipulative styles, with the difference that one neither attacks nor manipulates the other, because self-expression always occurs with respect for the other person. It is a win-win situation: Not only do I achieve my goal, but I also embrace yours, and together, eventually finding common ground, we each reach our own goals. The assertive style certainly implies a strong sense of self-efficacy, i.e. the objective, not devaluative, evaluation that each person makes of themselves, their abilities and their ability to achieve their goals. An assertive person also has good emotional intelligence because they are able to not only understand and express their own emotions but also understand and respect those of others. This person practises active and open listening, is willing to listen to others and changes their opinion if they recognize that the other person's perspective is better than their own. They resist manipulation, enjoy and seek positive discussion and collaboration and have fairly high self-esteem.

A recent study from the United States reveals that doctors frequently interrupt patients soon after initiating a consultation. Although open-ended questions, such as "What brings you here today?" are regarded as fundamental for patient-centred care, only about one-third of physicians begin visits this way. Even when they do, patients are typically given a median of merely 11 s to respond before being interrupted. Dr. Naykky Singh Ospina, an internist and faculty member at the University of Florida, emphasizes that patients need to feel genuinely heard in order to trust that their physician is there to help them. Her analysis of 112 recorded clinical encounters in Wisconsin and Minnesota demonstrates that family physicians tend to allow patients more time—an average of 19 s—while specialists, who often rely on prior referral notes, interrupt sooner. This practice, she argues, risks missing crucial details that patients might disclose if permitted to speak for as little as two uninterrupted minutes. The study [31], published in the *Journal of General Internal Medicine*, also notes that only a minority of physicians explicitly ask patients what outcomes they hope to achieve from the visit. Although some interruptions may be intended to clarify or focus a discussion, the brevity of patient speaking time reflects deeper systemic issues: time constraints, inadequate training in communication skills, physician burnout and the distracting demands of electronic medical records. Dr. Ospina insists that authentic dialogue is a cornerstone of patient-centred care and calls for further investigation into why such engagement is often lacking. Similar patterns are observed in Canada, where medical educators, such as Dr. Arno Kumagai of the University of Toronto, acknowledge that students are taught to elicit patient values and preferences early in their training, but this focus diminishes once they enter clinical environments shaped by fee-for-service models and institutional cultures that prioritize efficiency over conversation. Both experts argue that although the principles of listening can be taught, they must also be actively reinforced within the culture of medicine to ensure that patient narratives are not lost amid administrative pressures and clinical routines [32].

2.5 Communication with an Inclusive Gender Perspective

The language we use in our workplace in an increasingly interconnected and diverse world is not only a means of communication but also a powerful tool for inclusion and representation. Aware of this reality, many companies, cooperatives, social enterprises and public and private institutions are committed to promoting language that respects and values gender diversity and contributes to a fair and inclusive work environment for all. This manual was created to guide our organization's members in using language and communication methods that reflect the principles of gender equality and inclusion. Inclusive communication is essential not only to respect the dignity of each person but also to strengthen our company's identity and values, improving the quality of our interactions both internally and externally. I will seek to promote a greater awareness of gender equality and inclusion in this section, encouraging reflection on one's own communication habits to contribute to the creation of a more welcoming and respectful work environment, where each person feels valued and included. Gender equality and inclusion must not only be declared values, but principles actively practised in our daily communication. This is a fundamental step towards a cultural shift that begins with language and extends to all aspects of our business. But what do we mean by inclusive language?

Inclusive language is an approach to communication that aims to avoid exclusion, prejudice or discrimination, making all people visible and respected, regardless of their gender, age, origin, ability or any other characteristic. It is a conscious use of words and expressions that recognizes diversity and promotes equity. In the business context, this means choosing terms and linguistic constructions that include all the people who make up our work environment and the broader community with which we interact. For this reason, it is essential to give due weight to inclusive language for gender equality. Gender equality is a fundamental objective for society and the world of work and education. Language, as a tool for representing reality, plays a key role in this context. Inclusive language actively contributes to reducing gender stereotypes and promoting a culture of equality [33]. Through the use of language that reflects fairness and respect for all gender identities, we help create a work environment where each person feels recognized and valued. We can convey and reinforce stereotypes and prejudices through the written and spoken word, but we can also convey inclusivity. Gender-sensitive language was born precisely for this: a need and a right to include every person in spoken and written language, but it can often clash with grammatical rules, or sometimes, prejudices and conflicting opinions among "purists".

"A woman must have money and a room of her own if she is to write fiction", as Virginia Woolf wrote in her famous novel *A Room of One's Own* [34], but a woman also needs the freedom to express her thoughts through a language she can make her own and that allows her to be understood by others who share her language. The adoption of inclusive language has a significant impact on the corporate climate. It promotes a sense of belonging and respect among employees, creating a more positive and productive work environment. Furthermore, it reflects a modern and socially responsible image of our organization, strengthening the trust and respect of customers, partners and the public at large. Careful and inclusive communication is a hallmark of an organization that looks to the future, values diversity, and is committed to building a more just and equitable society. Gender-sensitive communication is often overlooked as a priority, yet it is precisely these small, everyday gestures that have helped change our society. These gestures will, sooner or later, become part of our way of communicating, up to the time they are fully integrated. Until we no longer speak of neutral language but simply of language. These guidelines aim to combat the prejudice associated with a typically patriarchal culture that struggles to include women, not only in language but also within society itself. Our communication must reflect gender balance, ensuring both genders are equally represented. This means alternating between feminine and masculine forms when referring to roles, professions or groups of people. It is important that both genders feel seen and included in our language. This practice goes beyond mere formal correctness; it reaffirms our commitment to an inclusive and respectful work environment. Whenever possible, it is advisable to use gender-neutral terms to avoid focusing on a specific gender. This can be particularly useful in situations where the person's gender is unknown or irrelevant. Instead of "chairman" or "chairwoman", for example, you can use "chairperson" or simply "president". This approach not only promotes gender equality but also simplifies communication, making it more direct and inclusive. Avoiding gender stereotypes is crucial in our communications. This includes avoiding associating specific characteristics, skills or interests exclusively with one gender. Assuming that all employees in a given sector are male or that all secretaries are female, for example, perpetuates outdated and limiting ideas. Instead, we must strive to represent people in a way that reflects the diversity and complexity of the real world. Images play as important a role as words in corporate communications. The images we choose to represent our organization can have a significant impact on the public's perception of our values and commitment to inclusion and diversity. An image can convey powerful messages, often more immediately and directly than text. Therefore, it is essential to choose images that reflect the diversity of our community and promote a balanced and inclusive image. The first step could be to use the double form (Mr. and Mrs.) in written communications, especially in emails within the company or with clients. One precaution we can take is to try, where possible, to use rewordings, such as "those who" and "the people who", finding a semantically neutral form. The choice of possible strategies among those suggested here must be carefully evaluated on a case-by-case basis. In any case, the important thing is to understand that language plays a fundamental role in the perception and construction of reality and identity. What we should aspire to is an inclusive society that values existing differences.

2.6 Creativity, Divergent Thinking and Problem-Solving Applied to the Pharmacy Context

Originally Edward de Bono related a story in *The Use of Lateral Thinking* called the "Tale of Two Pebbles". A farmer living in a small Indian village owed a great deal of money to the local moneylender. The latter was elderly and unattractive but lusted after the farmer's beautiful daughter. He suggested that the debt the farmer owed would be cancelled if the farmer's daughter became the moneylender's wife. The girl and her father were appalled by the idea. The clever moneylender proposed that fate decide the outcome. He said that he would place a white and a black pebble into a moneybag. The daughter would then pick one pebble out of the bag without looking. If the black pebble was chosen, the girl would marry the moneylender, and he would cancel the farmer's debt. If the white pebble was chosen, the moneylender would stay single and the debt the farmer owed would still be cancelled. While they were discussing this, the moneylender picked up two pebbles from the path on which they stood. The observant girl noticed that he had chosen two black pebbles, which he placed in the money bag. He then offered the bag to the girl to pick out a pebble. Imagine the situation. What would you do in her position? What would you have advised her to do? Think about it. The girl plucked a pebble out of the bag and, without looking at it, clumsily dropped it onto the path among hundreds of other pebbles. She apologised for her clumsiness but then pointed out that if the moneylender looked at the pebble remaining in the bag, he would know which one she had picked. The moneylender did not want to admit he had cheated. The girl had altered a seemingly terrible situation into a very good one.

Defined by Edward de Bono [35], lateral thinking refers to the ability to see situations and problems from different perspectives, breaking traditional thought patterns to find creative solutions. The term has roots in cognitive psychology and creativity theory and emphasizes the importance of mental flexibility and the ability to look beyond appearances. Practical examples include using metaphors to solve puzzles, brainstorming to generate original ideas and applying analogies to develop new solutions to existing problems, demonstrating how lateral thinking can be a powerful tool for innovating and improving processes in various contexts, from everyday life to professional challenges. Divergent thinking is a way of thinking that involves generating multiple creative solutions to a single problem, emphasizing originality and variety of ideas. Lateral thinking, on the other hand, focuses on reframing the problem itself, seeking new and unconventional perspectives to find innovative solutions. Both types of thinking share the characteristic of breaking traditional patterns and encouraging creativity but differ in their specific approaches and objectives. Divergent thinking is often used during the initial brainstorming phase, where the quantity of ideas is more important than their immediate application, while lateral thinking is used to reframe existing problems and find new solutions. Lateral thinking can be developed through a variety of techniques and strategies aimed at fostering creativity and mental flexibility.

Among the most effective techniques are brainstorming, which encourages the generation of a wide range of ideas without immediate judgement; role-playing, which allows you to view a problem from multiple perspectives; and the use of mind maps, which helps visualize connections between different ideas and concepts. Practical exercises such as solving puzzles, tackling problems with seemingly illogical solutions and breaking habitual thought patterns are also useful. Furthermore, the importance of creativity and mental flexibility cannot be underestimated: reading, exploring new interests and challenging one's beliefs are effective ways to foster lateral thinking. Creating an environment that encourages creative thinking and experimentation, without fear of failure, is crucial for developing lateral thinking in both education and the professional world. Edward de Bono's *Six Thinking Hats* [35] facilitates lateral thinking by offering six distinct ways of looking at things. Here is what they mean and what it means to wear them:

White hat: represents facts and objective information; wearing it means analysing available data without emotional influences or judgements

Red hat: represents emotions and intuitions; wearing it means expressing feelings and immediate reactions without the need for logical justification.

Black hat: represents critical thinking and judgment; wearing it means focusing on the risks, difficulties and critical aspects of a situation or idea.

Yellow hat: represents optimism and constructiveness; wearing it means seeking the benefits, opportunities and positive aspects of a situation or idea.

Green hat: represents creativity and innovation; wearing it means generating new ideas, alternative solutions and thinking outside the box.

Blue hat: represents control and organization of the thought process; wearing it means managing the thinking process, ensuring that the other hats are used effectively and in a coordinated manner.

Due to past experiences or fear, people often tend to wear only, or predominantly, the black hat, which keeps them safe from danger by analysing risks and critical issues. However, it is helpful to switch hats and experiment with multiple perspectives to gain a comprehensive and balanced vision, fostering creative and innovative solutions. This technique allows you to explore a problem from different angles, promoting a multidimensional and more flexible view of situations, an essential element for lateral thinking. The six thinking hats technique can be used in many everyday situations to improve the quality of decisions and solve problems more effectively.

Within the organizational context of the pharmacy, team meetings represent decisive moments for defining operational strategies, addressing critical issues and updating clinical protocols. The adoption of lateral thinking within these meetings makes it possible to broaden the range of potential solutions, fostering more deliberate and innovative decisions. Lateral thinking functions as a tool for multidimensional exploration. Rather than confining discussion to a strictly linear process, it encourages team members to consider unconventional perspectives. During a meeting focused on managing the stock of a medication with limited availability, for instance, the pharmacist might propose not only a revision of the supply plan but also temporary collaboration with neighbouring pharmacies or the introduction of already validated therapeutic substitution protocols. This approach broadens the spectrum of possibilities and leads the group to analyse options that, in a purely vertical context, would have remained unexplored. The practice of lateral thinking proves particularly effective when the team faces complex problems. A concrete example is the introduction of a new clinical service, such as the care pathway for chronically ill patients undergoing polypharmacy. Instead of approaching implementation as a single, monolithic task, lateral thinking guides the team to break the problem down into manageable components. The team might first define criteria for patient inclusion, then determine how to record clinical data, identify suitable digital tools for monitoring and plan the internal training of staff. This decomposition makes it possible to assign specific responsibilities, develop micro-solutions and approach the overall challenge in a systematic way, thereby reducing the complexity perceived and increasing the likelihood of success. Lateral thinking also stimulates creativity and leads to more effective solutions. During a meeting aimed at reducing waiting times at the counter, for example, pharmacists may be encouraged to explore unusual but potentially effective strategies, such as implementing a digital booking system for repeat prescriptions or creating dedicated time slots for specific services. This openness to out-of-the-box ideas, examined collectively and critically discussed, enables the team to reach decisions that balance innovation with feasibility. In conclusion, integrating lateral thinking into team meetings enables pharmacists and other staff members to navigate the inherent complexity of the field more effectively. Decisions not only become more carefully reasoned through the exploration of alternative perspectives, the systematic breakdown of challenges and the pursuit of creative solutions but also often lead to organizational practices that enhance the overall efficiency of the service.

2.7 Bystander Effect and Social Influence: The Otherness

How many times have we read or heard news reports of arguments, fights, episodes of violence or bullying in which no bystander intervened to help the victim? And how many times have we wondered why, in emergency situations, it is not instinctive to head towards the crisis and offer help rather than look around waiting to see what others are doing?

Many of us have probably responded to this question by thinking we were surrounded by insensitive, cowardly people who were not genuinely willing to lend a helping hand. Social psychology, however, has been studying this phenomenon for years, more accurately called the "bystander effect" (or bystander apathy). It reveals people's tendency not to intervene in emergency situations when others are present. Specifically, according to this effect, the greater the number of bystanders in an emergency situation, the less likely it is that someone will help/intervene. Social psychologists Bibb Latanè and John Darley [36] coined the name for this phenomenon and studied its causes and consequences. Their research stemmed from a murder that occurred in New York City one evening in 1964: A young woman, Catherine Susan "Kitty" Genovese, was returning home from work when she was suddenly attacked by a knife-wielding maniac. Initially, the young woman's loud screams and her attempts to defend herself repelled the attacker, but when the man saw no one coming to her aid, he decided to attack her again, this time sexually assaulting her, robbing her and stabbing her to death. During the half-hour it took the man to kill the girl, no one who lived nearby and witnessed the screams came to her aid. However, when the police questioned residents of the neighbourhood, 38 people admitted to hearing screams, and one of them directly testified to the incident. Each of them would have had the time they needed to do something, but they all remained trapped by inertia, refusing to act. Why? If it is understandable that a person would not go out into the street for fear of being attacked themselves, why had no one at least called the police?

Starting with their interest in the Genovese case, Darley and Latanè launched one of the most important research programmes in social psychology to date. The two first outlined the fundamental and distinctive elements of an emergency situation and agreed that it is an unusual and unexpected event; it can vary widely in nature; it can be dangerous; and it requires immediate action.

They then sought to understand whether empathy for the suffering of others or a minimal sense of civic responsibility was sufficient to induce people to intervene in dangerous situations, and they also asked whether the presence of other bystanders at a potential critical event was an incentive to provide help. A lack of intervention would undoubtedly be more easily justified and labelled as apathy, selfishness and insensitivity on the part of the bystander. However, the two scholars attempted to shift the focus to people's thought processes, hypothesizing that more rational processes were involved in this phenomenon. Specifically, it was found that a lack of help occurs more frequently when the number of witnesses to the event increases, while when only one bystander is present, the sense of responsibility increases and, consequently, the ability to act. Why does this happen? According to the cognitive model developed by Latanè and Darley, a person's help depends on the results of a series of decisions and psychological processes that can trigger a reluctance in people to intervene if other bystanders are present. These are not specific characteristics of individuals but rather dynamics established among witnesses. Three main processes are activated in these situations:

> Diffusion of responsibility: The presence of other people (even one is enough for this process to come into play) offers everyone the opportunity to transfer responsibility for action or inaction to them. A single person is much more likely to intervene to help the victim precisely because the victim perceives full responsibility for the action as their own.
>
> Pluralistic ignorance and social influence: This refers to the tendency of people to be guided by others regarding the most appropriate behaviour in a given context, believing that others have more information and the necessary skills to be able to help. Essentially, other witnesses serve as role models, and consequently, if they adopt a passive attitude, the emergency situation may seem less serious and urgent than it is, discouraging everyone from responding.
>
> Public inhibition: This is essentially the fear of making a bad impression in front of others, fearing that they might consider one's action-reaction excessive or inappropriate.

In short, it is as if the number of people increases, one feels protected by a sort of anonymity that diminishes the sense of personal responsibility and inhibits action. However, it has been observed that there are also cases in which some people are more inclined to intervene and provide assistance. In particular, it emerged that this occurs when the bystander knows the victim, when they believe the person in difficulty deserves help, when they have medical training/experience and are trained in self-defence and when the victim finds the strength to clearly point out one or more people present, asking for their help and investing them with an immediate sense of responsibility. The bystander effect can manifest itself even in the seemingly simplest situations of our daily lives and can unfortunately have truly dramatic consequences. For this reason, it is important to educate ourselves and be aware of this insidious phenomenon, the mechanisms that regulate it and its negative effects on society. We strive to counter it with courage, education, awareness and, above all, by working to embrace individual responsibility. Indeed, we are all responsible for what happens around us, and it is important to remember that every single action can truly make a difference in emergency situations. Personal responsibility and altruism are fundamental elements for creating a more supportive society and promoting a culture of intervention in which mutual aid and individual action are encouraged and valued. Only in this way can we break the cycle of the bystander effect and affirm the power of individual action in a predominantly observant society. Awareness of this dynamic is particularly significant for pharmacists. By virtue of their professional role, pharmacists frequently operate in community settings and are, therefore, among the first health professionals to encounter emergency situations. These may include sudden medical crises occurring within the pharmacy itself—such as anaphylactic reactions, seizures or cardiac events—or emergencies that arise in public spaces. In such contexts, the bystander effect poses a risk, as hesitation or reliance on others to act can delay critical interventions.

A pharmacist, however, is expected to transcend the bystander effect. This entails recognizing an emergency without waiting for others to take initiative and assuming personal responsibility for initiating appropriate measures. From a professional and ethical standpoint, pharmacists are bound by their status as healthcare providers to offer immediate assistance within the scope of their training. This includes activating emergency services without presuming that another person has already done so, and applying first aid competencies, such as those acquired through Basic Life Support training, in order to stabilize the individual while awaiting specialized help. Moreover, the pharmacist may be required to coordinate bystanders, providing clear instructions to ensure that assistance is both organized and effective. The importance of overcoming the bystander effect in pharmacy practice is twofold. Firstly, it is essential for safeguarding patient safety, as timely intervention can prevent deterioration and, in some cases, be life-saving. Secondly, it upholds the ethical and deontological principles that underpin the profession, reinforcing the public's trust in pharmacists as accessible and competent health professionals capable of responding decisively in critical situations.

2.8 Practice Time

1. What do you mean by the concept of care?
2. What are some of the most common interpretations of this concept?
3. What does the *Myth of Care* tell us, and why is it important?
4. What types of communication are you familiar with?
5. According to the scientists who discovered them, what is the function of mirror neurons?
6. What is the purpose of De Bono hats?
7. What is the bystander effect?

References

1. Preta L, Donghi P. In principio era la cura. Roma-Bari: Laterza; 1995.
2. Flecha R. Sharing words: theory and practice of dialogic learning. Lanham: University Press of America; 2000.
3. Vygotsky LS. Mind in society: development of higher psychological processes. Cambridge: Harvard University Press; 1978.
4. Freire P. Pedagogy of the oppressed. New York: Seabury Press; 1970.
5. Bruner J. The culture of education. Cambridge: Harvard University Press; 1996.
6. Habermas J. The theory of communicative action. Frankfurt am Main: Suhrkamp; 1981.
7. Austin JL. How to do things with words. Oxford: Oxford University Press; 1975.
8. Mead GH. Mind, self, and society from the standpoint of a social behaviorist. Chicago: University of Chicago Press; 1934.
9. Gadamer H-G. Hermeneutics and social science. Dordrecht: Reidel Publishing Company; 1975.
10. Mayeroff M. On caring. New York: Harper & Row; 1971.

11. Oxford Latin Dictionary [Internet]. Available from: https://www.oxfordscholarlyeditions.com/page/95.
12. Hanisch H. How care holds humanity: the myth of Cura and theories of care. Med Humanit. 2022;48:e1–9.
13. Heidegger M. Being and time. New ed. Oxford: Basil Blackwell; 1973.
14. Kleinman A, van der Geest S. 'Care' in health care: remaking the moral world of medicine. Med Anthropol. 2009;21(1):159–68.
15. Kristeva J, Moro MR, Ødemark J, Engebretsen E. Cultural crossings of care: an appeal to the medical humanities. Med Humanit. 2018;44(1):55–8.
16. Burdach K. Faust und die Sorge. Dtsch Vierteljahrsschr Literaturwiss Geistesgesch. 1923;1:160.
17. Seneca. Epistulae morales ad Lucilium, vol. 3. Gummere RM, translator. Cambridge: Harvard University Press; 1953.
18. Charon J-E. L'Esprit, cet Inconnu. Paris: Albin Michel; 1977.
19. MacDougall D. Hypothesis concerning soul substance toegther with experimental evidence of such a substance. J Am Soc Psych Res. 1907;1(5):237.
20. Von Goethe JW. Goethe's Faust. Kaufmann W, translator. New York: Vintage; 1962.
21. Herder JG. Das Kind der Sorge. In: Gaier U, editor. Herders Werke, vol. 3. Berlin: Deutscher Klassiker Verlag; 1990.
22. Kierkegaard S, Consider the lilies: being the second part of "edifying discourses in a different vein". Aldworth ASF, translator, Ferrie AS. London: C. W. Daniel; 1940.
23. Goleman D. Emotional intelligence. New York: Bantam Books; 1995.
24. Levenson RW, Ruef AM. Empathy: a physiological substrate. J Pers Soc Psychol. 1992;63(2):234–46.
25. Damasio AR. The feeling of what happens: body and emotion in the making of consciousness. New York: Harcourt Brace; 1999.
26. Poli EF. Le emozioni che curano. Milano: Mondadori; 2020.
27. Rizzolatti G, Sinigaglia C. Mirroring brains: how we understand others from inside. Oxford: Oxford University Press; 2023.
28. Candace B. Molecules of emotion: the science between mind-body medicine. New York: Scribner; 1999.
29. May R. Love and will. New York: W.W. Norton & Company; 1969.
30. Watzlawick P, Beavin Bavelas J, Jackson DD, O'Hanlon B. Pragmatics of human communication: a study of interactional patterns, pathologies and paradoxes. New York: Norton & Co; 1978.
31. Ospina NS, Phillips KA, Rodriguez-Gutierrez R, Castaneda-Guerderas A, Gionfriddo MR, Branda ME, Montori VM. Eliciting the patient's agenda—secondary analysis of recorded clinical encounters. J Gen Intern Med. 2019;34(1):36–40.
32. Noakes S. If the doctor is listening, you have 11 seconds. CBC News [Internet] 2018 Jul 23. Available from: https://www.cbc.ca/news/health/doctor-patient-visits-1.4755498.
33. European Commission. European Commission campaign against gender stereotypes [Internet]. Available from: https://end-gender-stereotypes.campaign.europa.eu/index_it.
34. Woolf V. A room of one's own. London: Hogarth Press; 1929.
35. De Bono E. The use of lateral thinking. London: Jonathan Cape; 1967.
36. Latanè B, Darley J. The unresponsive bystander: why doesn't he help? Englewood Cliffs: Prentice Hall; 1970.

Chapter 3
Pharmacy in Intercultural Contexts and in Educational and Cultural Inequalities

3.1 Introduction

Gaps in care are closely linked to multiple forms of inequality that affect the well-being of unpaid caregivers and care recipients alike. In such contexts, a person may be living in what Kröger terms "care poverty", a condition in which essential care needs remain unmet due to systemic shortcomings rather than individual circumstances [1]. The concept of care poverty highlights situations of structural failure, emphasizing that access to care is not merely a matter of personal vulnerability, such as age or disability, but is shaped more by institutional, economic and social factors that limit the availability and adequacy of both formal services and informal networks [2]. These structural barriers mean that individuals in lower-income households, marginalized communities or regions with weaker service infrastructures experience a disproportionate burden, deepening existing inequalities in health, autonomy and overall quality of life. Furthermore, beyond the immediate health and well-being of home-care clients and caregivers, these gaps carry significant economic implications. Recent work on the care economy demonstrates that the provision of social and material care, whether paid or unpaid, is fundamental to broader economic functioning [3]. When care systems fail, the resulting unpaid labour, financial strain and lost workforce participation are not evenly distributed; instead, they reinforce and exacerbate social and gender inequalities. Women, who make up the majority of unpaid caregivers, are particularly affected, often facing reduced earnings, stalled careers and increased vulnerability to poverty. In this way, care poverty does not merely reflect a lack of services, it represents a structural driver of inequity, perpetuating cycles of disadvantage within families and across generations.

S. Leoncini, *The Relationship between Pharmacists and Patients*, New Paradigms in Healthcare, https://doi.org/10.1007/978-3-032-21249-8_3

3.2 Illiteracy, Socio-economic Hardship, Refugees and Migrants: Stereotypes and Prejudice

Social and economic inequalities represent one of the most complex and urgent challenges in today's global context, and they also have repercussions in the healthcare sector. Healthcare systems are called upon to meet an unprecedented demand for equity and access to care in a world marked by growing fragility and persistent phenomena of exclusion. A significant portion of the population, in fact, lives in conditions of pronounced vulnerability: Individuals lacking adequate economic resources, living in unstable family and social environments or residing in marginal areas face structural and cultural barriers in obtaining treatments, medications and essential services.

No pandemic in the last century, despite several significant outbreaks, has produced consequences as devastating as those of COVID-19. Its impact was not only lethal for public health but also profoundly disruptive to economic systems, education, communication and virtually every dimension of social life. The Spanish flu of 1918–1919 caused a far greater number of deaths: estimates range from 20 to 50 million worldwide. However, that event unfolded in a world entirely different from ours; one already exhausted by a global conflict and lacking even the most basic healthcare infrastructures. The third wave of that flu, which proved to be the most lethal, struck during the winter of 1919, when viral pneumonias were compounded by bacterial infections for which antibiotics were not yet available. This raises a crucial question: How could an infectious outbreak in the third millennium, within societies as technologically advanced as ours, exert such a devastating effect on social relations and well-being?

A compelling answer lies in the concept of a syndemic. This term, a synthesis of "synergy", "epidemic", "pandemic" and "endemic", coined by medical anthropologist Merrill Singer in the 1990s [4, 5], refers to the compounded negative effects on individuals and societies generated by the synergistic interaction of two or more diseases. The syndemics model of health centres on the concept of a biosocial complex, understood as the dynamic interplay of coexisting or sequential diseases and the social and environmental conditions that foster and intensify the detrimental effects of their interaction. This emerging perspective on health and clinical practice challenges the traditional view of diseases as discrete, self-contained entities, isolated from one another and independent of the social contexts in which they arise. Instead, the syndemics framework highlights the ways in which biological and social factors intersect and act synergistically, producing significant consequences for both individual and population health.

More specifically, a syndemic approach investigates:

- Why certain diseases tend to cluster within individuals and communities
- The biological pathways through which these conditions interact and amplify the overall burden of disease
- How social environments, particularly settings marked by inequality and injustice, shape patterns of clustering, interaction and vulnerability

Within this series, particular attention is devoted to the contributions of the syndemics paradigm in elucidating the interactions among chronic diseases in their social context, as well as the implications of adopting a syndemics perspective for advancing health rights. In the case of COVID-19, the pandemic interacted with another, more insidious global health crisis: the escalating prevalence of chronic diseases. Over the past four decades, particularly since the 1980s, cardiovascular diseases, cancers, obesity and diabetes have accelerated dramatically across all regions of the globe. The destructive effects of this syndemic became evident from the earliest phases of COVID-19 when mortality rates were shown to be disproportionately high among populations burdened by chronic illnesses. Statistical analyses in the United States, for example, revealed that African American populations experienced mortality rates approximately double those of white populations, owing to both a higher prevalence of chronic conditions and greater exposure to infection due to occupational and housing factors. Similar patterns of inequality have been observed elsewhere, and it is likely that detailed studies in other countries will reveal a comparable widening of health disparities. The strain on healthcare systems was immediate and severe. Both infectious outbreaks and chronic disease epidemics require strong frontline defences: effective preventive measures, early detection and timely intervention to avert complications. This demands robust community-based healthcare services, including primary care networks and public health infrastructures. Over time, however, many of these systems have been eroded. The absence of effective territorial "filters"—family physicians, public health services and preventive networks—have left populations disoriented and overwhelmed hospitals with cases that might otherwise have been managed in the community. Understanding the causes of these converging pandemics is more complex. Yet one striking observation emerges: both phenomena have roots traceable to human behaviour and decisions over recent decades. In the realm of chronic disease, profound transformations in dietary habits and food systems have occurred. These changes stem from an intricate interplay of socio-cultural, environmental and economic factors: rapid urbanization, shifts in family structures, reduced time devoted to home cooking, widening socio-economic inequalities and, crucially, the aggressive expansion of global food and beverage industries. Multinational corporations have played a central role in accelerating the nutritional transition from traditional diets to those dominated by highly processed foods and sugar-laden beverages. These products, often termed unhealthy commodities, are characterized by a low nutritional value, high caloric density and excessive sugar or salt content, contributing substantially to the worldwide surge in chronic diseases, a true industrial epidemic. Similarly, human activity is implicated in the origins of COVID-19 itself [6]. Quammen underscores that human encroachment on ecosystems through deforestation, habitat disruption and the mixing of previously isolated species creates unprecedented opportunities for viral transmission. Such spillover events can rapidly escalate in an interconnected world of over seven billion potential hosts, magnified by global travel and trade.

Ultimately, the syndemic of COVID-19 reflects a convergence of biological and social processes shaped by human action. Understanding this interplay is not only an academic exercise but a prerequisite for designing more resilient health systems, addressing structural inequalities and preventing future global crises. In this context, the role of pharmacists assumes a strategic significance and, in certain respects, an even more incisive impact compared to other healthcare professionals. Their contribution goes well beyond the mere dispensing of medicines; they perform a complex function of mediation, guidance and support aimed at ensuring that even individuals in situations of extreme vulnerability can access appropriate treatments. Their work is, therefore, configured not merely as a technical-professional service but as a safeguard of equity and social justice, making a significant contribution to reducing the impact of inequalities on public health while also challenging stereotypes and prejudice. In common perception, discrimination is often considered a phenomenon confined to specific social strata, particularly those that are less educated or economically disadvantaged. However, sociological and psychological research has demonstrated that stereotypes and prejudices cut across all social classes, including those that are economically privileged and culturally advantaged, where one would expect a more critical, open and respectful approach towards others. Gordon Allport observes that prejudice is an aversive or hostile attitude towards a person who belongs to a group, simply because he or she belongs to that group, and is, therefore, presumed to have the objectionable qualities ascribed to the group [7]. Stereotypes, on the other hand, represent a different level of analysis. According to Aronson and colleagues, stereotypes are cognitive schemas that simplify and organize information about people based on their membership in social categories [8, p. 412]. A stereotype is, thus, a rigid and oversimplified belief, often transmitted culturally and rarely questioned. It can be either positive or negative, but, in any case, it reduces the complexity of the other to a few characteristics. Prejudice is the affective and evaluative consequence of such simplification: it does not merely involve stereotypical thinking but entails a value judgment (often negative) and a predisposition to discriminate. Henri Tajfel explains that stereotypes provide a cognitive justification for our affective reactions of prejudice, and these reactions are then rationalized as if they were based on factual evidence [9]. The presence of these cognitive mechanisms is not limited to relations between majorities and ethnic minorities, nor to gender relations. They permeate every sphere of social life: They can manifest as invisible barriers in the workplace, in educational pathways, in access to healthcare services and even in everyday interpersonal interactions. Particularly insidious is that form of discrimination which leaves no material trace but gradually undermines a person's self-esteem and dignity, as in the case of psychological or economic violence. Such dynamics, difficult to detect, represent "a mirror of the hierarchies present in our society" [10, p. 35] and are nourished precisely by unchallenged stereotypes. Preventing discrimination and prejudice entails creating spaces of care—educational, physical and symbolic—that foster critical reflection and the deconstruction of dominant representations. It is necessary to encourage the freedom to transgress imposed models and open one's gaze to the plurality of individual identities. The experiences of migrants, for example, demonstrate that identity is not a static entity but a dynamic process in constant redefinition, in which the culture of origin, age, social class, educational trajectory and the context of reception intertwine to generate new forms of subjectivity [11]. These reflections have tangible implications in the professional realm as well. The risk of being guided by stereotypes and prejudices is ever-present in the healthcare sector and particularly in the daily practice of pharmacists: A patient's physical appearance, manner of speaking, clothing or place of origin can trigger distorted initial impressions. Tajfel reminds us that first impressions are often distorted by pre-existing social categories [9]. For this reason, pharmacists must consciously move beyond such impressions and stereotypes, systematically gathering information, listening attentively and respecting each patient's specificity. Only in this way is it possible to ensure a truly effective service grounded in professional ethics, preventing clinical or communicative decisions from being influenced by unconscious biases. Ultimately, the challenge is to cultivate a critical capacity that enables the recognition of stereotypes and prejudices in oneself and others, thereby transforming every relationship of care, education, professional practice and social interaction into an opportunity to move beyond appearances and engage with the full complexity of each individual.

3.3 Disability: The Biopsychosocial Perspective

The WHO developed the International Classification of Functioning, Disability and Health (ICF) as a conceptual framework designed to describe health and disability in a systematic and standardized way [12, 13]. The ICF is far more than a simple list of diseases; it introduces a shared language and an interpretative structure that allow health professionals to consider a person's health condition in its entirety, including the complex interplay between biological, psychological and social factors. Unlike the traditional individual-medical model, which tends to interpret illness merely as a set of deficits inherent to the individual, the ICF proposes a biopsychosocial approach. This perspective emphasizes the dynamic interaction between personal characteristics and environmental contexts. In doing so, it moves beyond a merely deficit-oriented and reductionist view of illness, fostering a more nuanced, less stigmatizing understanding of health conditions. This conceptual framework proves especially significant within healthcare settings and particularly in the practice of pharmacy. The pharmacist is not simply a dispenser of treatments; rather, they occupy a strategic position in the patient's care pathway and the therapeutic relationship itself. Viewing the individual not merely as a "bearer of disease" but as a person living with a specific condition within a particular environment enables the professional to establish a more empathetic and constructive relationship. It is important to note that hospital pharmacists, unlike community pharmacists, often work with patients affected by chronic conditions—individuals who may live for many years, or even an entire lifetime, with their disease. This clinical reality makes it even more relevant to adopt a model that accounts for functional capacities, contextual limitations and available resources, rather than focusing solely on pathophysiology. Adopting the ICF model, therefore, implies that pharmacists must cultivate communication and relational skills oriented towards recognizing the complexity of human functioning. This entails interpreting not only medical prescriptions but also the patient's expressed and unexpressed needs while taking into account the barriers and resources present in the patient's living environment. A patient with a chronic disease, for instance, is not defined solely by symptoms or clinical test results but also by everyday challenges, family support networks, work-related circumstances and environmental factors that all influence their quality of life. From this perspective, the pharmacist's role emerges as that of a skilled mediator between scientific knowledge and the patient's subjective experience. The aim is neither to judge a disease nor to rigidly categorize an individual but to initiate a dialogue that considers the functional dimensions described by the ICF: body functions and structures, activities and participation, and environmental and personal factors. Furthermore, applying the ICF model within the pharmaceutical field helps guide professional interventions towards more inclusive practices. Interaction with people affected by chronic conditions or disabilities cannot be reduced to technical communication alone; it must also include active listening skills, a readiness to clarify doubts and an openness to perceive subtle signs of difficulty, even when these are not explicitly stated. In this sense, the pharmacist becomes a promoter of a person-centred approach, where the act of dispensing a medication is integrated into a broader relational process aimed at supporting autonomy and overall well-being. The ICF, therefore, not only offers a common language for describing diverse health conditions but also serves as a valuable educational and operational tool for health professionals, including pharmacists, who are constantly confronted with the complexity of care [14, 15]. Ultimately, integrating the biopsychosocial model into pharmaceutical practice promotes a non-reductionist vision of illness, valuing the patient as an active subject rather than as a mere recipient of therapeutic prescriptions.

3.4 The Zone of Proximal Development

Every function in a child's cultural development manifests itself twice, or on two distinct levels. Initially, it appears at the social level and, subsequently, at the psychological level. At first, these functions are observed in interpersonal interactions, serving as interpsychological categories. This dual manifestation applies equally to voluntary attention, logical memory, concept formation and the development of willpower. The notion of the zone of proximal development (ZPD) indicates that psychological development can be directed externally, through guided interaction and scaffolding. Building on these foundational ideas, Piotr Galperin [16], one of Lev Vygotsky's [17] most devoted followers, emphasized the crucial role of the adult in teaching the child how to navigate problem-solving tasks. According to him, the child becomes consciously aware of the most effective strategies to employ only by actively guiding the child through the orientation process of a task. This awareness, in turn, enables the child to transfer the learned skills to analogous situations, thereby acting autonomously. This form of guided instruction is intimately connected to the necessity of fostering metacognitive activity, which serves as a guarantee for truly developmental and progressive learning. Following the concepts mentioned previously, it becomes clear that development is best understood as the outcome of a complex interaction between internal psychological processes and external environmental influences, realized through activity and communication. It is important to highlight that, while the psychological aspect is recognized as being shaped by living conditions and educational experiences, the internal psychological sphere itself maintains a relative degree of independence—a form of self-movement. This intrinsic autonomy ensures that individuals remain active agents, even capable of transforming the reality around them. Therefore, a key indicator of development lies in the capacity for self-regulation of behaviour, as well as in the development of formations related to self-awareness, including self-esteem and metacognition. The following theses can be inferred from this theoretical framework, grounded in Vygotskian understanding of the relationship between education and development:

- Development is the product of the assimilation of historical and social experience, which occurs through activity and communication.
- The principle of psychic formation results from the internalization of external actions that serve a guiding function; consequently, this process can be facilitated and directed by adults.
- Teaching functions as a guiding force that directs development, which should not be oriented towards past achievements but to the immediate future.
- The role of others, both adults and peers, is crucial for the intellectual development of children.
- It is essential to consider the level of support a child may require during the learning process.

Why is this understanding particularly important when working professionally with patients suffering from a wide range of pathologies? Within the context of the therapeutic relationship, knowledge of developmental and learning theories is crucial for ensuring the quality of professional interventions. Among these, Vygotsky's theory of the ZPD is particularly relevant, as it provides a conceptual framework for guiding patients in the process of understanding their clinical condition. Vygotsky defines the ZPD as the distance between the actual developmental level, determined by the ability to solve problems independently, and the level of potential development that can be achieved through guidance from an adult or collaboration with more competent peers [17]. Applied to healthcare settings, this perspective highlights that the patient is not a passive recipient of information but, instead, possesses prior knowledge, personal representations of illness and cognitive and emotional resources that can be activated through appropriately mediated interventions. A healthcare professional, who is aware of this dynamic, can adapt their language, provide clear and progressively structured explanations and create a relational context that functions as scaffolding—a temporary framework that supports the patient until they are able to comprehend and manage their condition more autonomously [18]. This approach is particularly significant because many patients lack prior medical knowledge and may experience illness with feelings of fear, anxiety or confusion [19]. In this sense, Vygotsky's theory enables professionals to interpret the educational-therapeutic process as a form of accompaniment: a path in which the patient is guided towards an understanding of their health status and treatments through communication that builds on their initial competencies and fosters further development. Such an approach not only promotes greater adherence to treatment but also enhances the patient's sense of self-efficacy and strengthens the trust within the clinician-patient relationship [20].

3.5 The Pygmalion Effect

Pygmalion, having seen how many women lived lives of shame,
horrified by those countless vices that nature had given to the female sex,
chose to remain unmarried and for a long time lived without a wife,
without a companion to share his bed.
But one day, with unmatched skill, he carved from bright ivory
a statue to which he gave a beauty no real woman could possess.
And he fell in love with his own work.
Her appearance was that of a living girl: you would have said she was about to move,
if modesty had not held her still;
so much artistry was hidden within the art.
Pygmalion was enchanted and felt his heart burn with passion for that lifeless form.
He would often run his hand over her, to test whether she was flesh or ivory,
and would not believe she was only ivory.
He kissed her, imagining she would return his kisses, he spoke to her, embraced her,
and thought he felt his fingers sink into her skin,
fearing even that he might bruise her.
He showered her with gifts that please young girls: seashells, smooth pebbles, little birds,
flowers of many colors, lilies, painted balls, amber tears from the trees of the Heliades.
Then he dressed her in fine garments, placed rings on her fingers, necklaces at her throat,
pearls in her ears, ribbons on her breast;
everything suited her, yet even bare she was most beautiful.
He laid her on couches dyed with Tyrian purple
and called her his companion, resting her head on soft pillows,
as if she could truly feel.
Meanwhile came the festival of Venus, most solemn in Cyprus:
heifers with golden horns were sacrificed, incense smoked on the altars.
Pygmalion, after making his offering, timidly said:
"O gods, if you can grant all things, give me as a wife…"
(he did not dare to say "my ivory maiden")
"…a woman like my ivory one."
Venus, present at her own feast, understood the prayer and, as a sign of her favor,
made the altar's flame leap up three times, bright and clear.
When he returned home, Pygmalion hurried to his statue,
bent over and kissed her: she seemed warm to the touch.
Again he felt her, caressed her breast:
the ivory lost its hardness, softened, yielded to his fingers,

> like Hymettian wax warmed by the sun and molded by a thumb,
> ready to take on many shapes, fit for the artist's hand.
> Amazed, wavering between joy and fear of being deceived,
> he touched again and again that dream that had become real: it was a living body!
> Veins throbbed beneath his thumb.
> Then the young man of Paphos poured out thanks to Venus,
> and at last pressed his lips to lips no longer false.
> The maiden felt his kisses, blushed, and, lifting timid eyes to the light,
> saw the sky, and saw, with it, the man who loved her. [21]

Robert Rosenthal and Lenore Jacobson conducted a landmark experiment in an American elementary school in the 1960s to evaluate the impact of teachers' expectations on students' academic performance [22]. The findings demonstrated a clear influence of expectations on intellectual achievements: The level attained by the students depended significantly on the beliefs and attitudes of their teachers. This phenomenon, known as the Pygmalion effect, the self-fulfilling prophecy or the Rosenthal effect, refers to a form of psychological suggestion through which an individual tends to adapt and conform their behaviour in line with the image, either positive or negative, that they hold in their own mind and perceive in the minds of others. The Pygmalion effect has been widely discussed and documented in various fields, particularly within psychology and pedagogy, and in medical-clinical settings, it resonates with the well-established concept of the placebo effect. A placebo is a substance commonly used in clinical trials as a control, devoid of any active pharmacological ingredients. The term "placebo effect" refers to the beliefs and expectations following the administration of such an inert substance: patients, convinced of the remedy's efficacy, report or experience improvements in health despite the absence of any active drug. Within healthcare contexts, the Pygmalion effect may also emerge in the relationship between healthcare professionals and their patients. The expectations held by clinicians, whether positive or negative, can subtly influence the course of care and patients' motivation to adhere to treatments or adopt lifestyle changes. When a physician underestimates a patient's ability to recover from a chronic condition, for instance, this implicit skepticism may be communicated, leading the patient to disengage and show a lower adherence to therapy. Conversely, overestimating a patient's resilience may result in overlooked warning signs or unaddressed needs, ultimately compromising the quality of care. A deeper understanding of the Pygmalion effect and its implications can, therefore, support more balanced therapeutic relationships and improve clinical outcomes.

3.6 Practice Time

1. What is the difference between pandemic and syndemic?
2. What is the ICF perspective?
3. Why is the ZPD particularly important when working professionally with patients suffering from a wide range of pathologies?
4. What do you mean by the concept of the Pygmalion effect?

References

1. Kröger T. Care poverty: unmet care needs in a Nordic welfare state. Int J Care Caring. 2022;6(1):123–47.
2. Kröger T, Leinonen A, Häikiö L. Care poverty in a Nordic welfare state: conceptual development and empirical evidence. Int J Sociol Soc Policy. 2019;39(3/4):221–34.
3. Peng I. The care economy, gender and inclusive growth in China. Int Labour Rev. 2018;157(4):609–30.
4. Singer M, Bulled N, Ostrach B, Mendenhall E. Syndemics and the biosocial conception of health. Lancet. 2017;389(10072):941–50.
5. Heidegger M. Being and time. Oxford: Basil Blackwell; 1973.
6. Quammen D. Spillover: animal infections and the next human pandemic offers a prophetic exploration of this dynamic. New York: W.W. Norton & Company; 2013.
7. Allport G. The nature of prejudice. Boston: Addison Wesley Publishing Company; 1954.
8. Aronson E, Wilson TD, Akert RM, Sommers SR. Social psychology. 9th ed. London: Pearson Education; 2019.
9. Tajfel H. Human groups and social categories. Studies in social psychology. Cambridge: Cambridge University Press; 1981.
10. Bourdieu P. La domination masculine. Paris: Éditions du Seuil; 1998.
11. Rutherford J, editor. Identity: community, culture, difference. London: Lawrence & Wishart; 1990.
12. World Health Organization. International classification of functioning, disability and health (ICF) [Internet]. Geneva: WHO; 2025 [cited 2025 Jul 25]. Available from: https://icd.who.int/browse/latest-release/icf/en.
13. World Health Organization. World Health Assembly resolution WHA 54.21: towards a common language for functioning, disability and health – endorsed 22 May 2001. In: International classification of functioning, disability and health [Internet]. Geneva: WHO; 2001 [cited 2025 Jul 25]. Available from: https://www.who.int/standards/classifications/international-classification-of-functioning-disability-and-health.
14. Stucki G, Ewert T, Cieza A, Bickenbach J, Chatterji S, Kostanjsek N, et al. ICF Core sets for chronic conditions. Disabil Rehabil. 2007;29(17):1141–7.
15. Üstün BT, Kostanjsek N, Chatterji S, Rehm J. WHO's ICF and functional status information in primary care. BMJ. 2006;333(7576):1215–6.
16. Galperin PY. Organization of mental activity and the effectiveness of learning. J Russ East Eur Psychol. 1992;30(4):65–82.
17. Vygotsky LS. Mind in society: development of higher psychological processes. Cambridge, MA: Harvard University Press; 1978.
18. Street RL Jr, Makoul G, Arora NK, Epstein RM. How does communication heal? Pathways linking clinician-patient communication to health outcomes. Patient Educ Couns. 2009;74(3):295–301.
19. Wood D, Bruner JS, Ross G. The role of tutoring in problem solving. J Child Psychol Psychiatry. 1876;17(2):89–100.
20. Borrel-Carrió F, Suchman AL, Epstein RM. The biopsychosocial model 25 years later: principles, practice, and scientific inquiry. Ann Fam Med. 2004;2(6):576–82.
21. Ovid. Metamorphoses. Book X, vv. 243–97.
22. Rosenthal R, Jacobson L. Pygmalion in the classroom: teacher expectation and pupils' intellectual development. New York: Holt, Rinehart & Winston; 1968.

Chapter 4
Self-Care

4.1 Introduction

Self-care has emerged in contemporary health discourse as a multifaceted concept that transcends the boundaries of medicine, psychology, philosophy and sociology. No longer limited to the mere management of minor ailments or the autonomous use of over-the-counter products, self-care today encompasses a broader set of practices aimed at maintaining physical, emotional and social well-being across the entire lifespan. It is an evolving construct, shaped by cultural, economic and technological factors, and one that calls for an interdisciplinary approach in both theoretical reflection and practical application. This chapter offers a comprehensive exploration of self-care, beginning with its conceptual foundations and continuing through its various manifestations in different stages of life, from early childhood to adulthood. Special attention is given to the aesthetic dimension of self-care, particularly through the use of cosmetics and beauty practices, which, far from being superficial, play a significant role in the construction of identity and self-esteem. At the same time, the chapter does not neglect the darker sides of self-management, such as the misuse of psychotropic medications, illegal substances and the development of addiction, phenomena that challenge the very idea of self-determination and personal autonomy. Finally, attention is turned to healthcare professionals themselves, with a focus on the risk of burnout among pharmacists. As intermediaries between patients and the healthcare system, pharmacists are increasingly called upon to not only support patients in their self-care journeys but also safeguard their own mental and emotional resilience. Through this multifocal lens, the chapter aims to offer a critical and integrated understanding of self-care as both an individual responsibility and a collective challenge.

S. Leoncini, *The Relationship between Pharmacists and Patients*, New Paradigms in Healthcare, https://doi.org/10.1007/978-3-032-21249-8_4

4.2 An Interdisciplinary Theory of Self-Care

The idea that one must dedicate time and attention to oneself, engaging in the care of the self, is currently a central theme in all professions of care, including teaching, medicine, nursing, pharmacy, social work and professional education. Yet the origins of this notion are deeply rooted in ancient Greek culture. Socrates, for instance, presents himself in Apology as a teacher of self-care, claiming before the judges that it is the deity who sent him to remind men not to be concerned with wealth or honour, but rather with themselves and their souls [1]. Subsequent philosophical traditions resumed and progressively placed at the centre of their inquiry what they considered the "art of existence", a form of living philosophy. The care of the self became a principle of general significance—transcending disciplinary boundaries and becoming a social practice. Michel Foucault regarded philosophy itself as a continuous exercise in the care of the self ([2] p. 46). Epicurus expressed a similar view in his "Letter to Menoeceus", asserting that "neither let the young delay in philosophizing, nor the old grow weary of it. One is never too young or too old for the health of the soul" ([2] p. 46]). Seneca, too, emphasized the necessity of constant self-reflection, writing, "He who wishes to be saved must live by constantly taking care of himself" [3]. Foucault reconstructs a precise and nuanced genealogy of this concept in his influential work "The care of the self", highlighting its persistent relevance. The French philosopher writes:

> The intensity of one's relationship with oneself – the forms in which one is called to take oneself as an object of knowledge and a field of action, with the goal of transforming, correcting, purifying oneself, and constructing one's own salvation. ([2] p. 46)

This reflection aligns with Hannah Arendt's exploration of the human condition. She analyses the fundamental human activities of labour, work and action in *The Human Condition* and how these shape human freedom and political life [4]. While Arendt does not explicitly use the term "care of the self" in the traditional Stoic or Nietzschean sense, her conception of political action presupposes a form of self-care grounded in public responsibility and ethical engagement. Action, according to Arendt, requires the ability to take a stance, articulate one's thoughts and act responsibly in the presence of others, thereby contributing to the creation and preservation of a shared world. In this sense, care of the self is intimately linked to the capacity for political responsibility and civic participation. For Arendt, human existence is always situated within the world; labour, work and action are the three fundamental activities that define our being-in-the-world. Labour sustains both individual survival and the life of the species. Work and its resulting human artefacts offer a measure of permanence in the face of life's transience and time's impermanence. Action, by contrast, establishes and maintains political communities and makes remembrance—history—itself possible. These activities are all rooted in natality, as they serve to prepare and preserve the world for new arrivals, who come into it as strangers. This naturally leads to the question: Was there truly no distinction between world and work in the ancient world? Was human occupation motivated primarily by the care of private matters or public ones?

4.2.1 *The Myth of Cronos and the Care of the Self*

There was once a blessed age for humankind, a time when the gods themselves took care of human beings. During that era, the god Cronos accompanied the universe in its motion: things came into being spontaneously, benefiting human life. Cronos, indeed, governed the circular movement of the cosmos by caring for the whole; the universe was divided into zones, each governed by a deity according to a singular principle of cosmic order. However, this state of blessedness, wherein human beings were recipients of divine care, was temporally limited. Once the time had reached its fulfilment and the movement of the cosmos attained its proper measure, Cronos withdrew to an external vantage point, outside the world's motion, and left it free. All other gods similarly abandoned the zones they had overseen. As a result, the cosmic movement no longer followed its original order, and human beings found themselves forsaken, no longer receiving divine care. Initially, being without tools or techniques, humans encountered significant hardships, especially with the cessation of spontaneous nourishment. Later, they received the gift of the techniques necessary for human life from the gods, through which they began to provide care for themselves.

Through this myth, we come to understand the human condition: From birth to death, human beings are no longer protected by divine care and are, thus, called to assume responsibility for self-care. Although we live in time, we hold no sovereignty over it. Unlike animals or plants, we are called to trace meaningful paths through existence. Our being, and thus the care for that being, is a constant process of becoming. This becoming is not merely a flow through time but a state of being entirely absorbed in the concern for existence [5].

Plato, through this myth, also warns us not to become selfish or overly self-focused. We are intrinsically relational beings; therefore, care of the self must proceed in tandem with care for the world and for others. It is precisely in caring for others that we discover our humanity, through a care for life that is inseparable from care for both ourselves and others. Following in the path of Socrates, the pursuit of knowledge and guiding others in this discovery does not consist in transmitting ready-made knowledge but remaining aware of the primacy of existence itself. Education, then, must consist in providing young people with experiences that awaken the desire to learn the practices necessary to pursue what is essential for rendering one's time authentic. In this sense, we cultivate a passion for self-formation that guides individuals in realizing their values [6].

The myth also teaches that becoming subjects of one's existence entails the decision to take responsibility for one's ontological weight to avoid letting time pass without shaping the direction of one's life. This inevitably involves moments of existential restlessness. The essential distinction here is that, through care of the self, we move from mere living, in which time is passively endured, to existence proper, in which life is formed according to specific desires and intentions. Epicurus, in his "Letter to Menoeceus" ([7] p. 122), argues that each human being must care for the soul continuously, devoting attention to it in every moment of every day.

Aristotle, in the *Nicomachean Ethics* [8], holds that we must strive for that which enhances life, which is truly good. Wisdom is not innate but rather an orientation of the soul nourished by the search for the good, understood as the ethical virtue of the soul. Part of this process of care also involves listening attentively to our affective experiences, which reveal our being in the here and now [9]. Martin Heidegger notes [10] that emotional attunement constitutes a fundamental existential phenomenon of human experience, as we are always immersed in emotions that shape the quality of our lives. Building on this, it is essential to interpret emotional experience by attributing to it a core of cognitive substance [11].

4.2.2 On the Distinction Between Caring About and Caring For

Traditional gender roles in our society imply that men care about and women care for. We often say in everyday language that we care for or about something or someone. A distinction can be drawn between "caring about" and "caring for", based on the nature of the object to which care is directed. "Caring about" generally refers to more abstract or less tangible objects and is marked by a broader, more generalized form of concern or commitment. By contrast, "caring for" implies a concrete, specific object and involves direct, often sustained attention to that object's needs. Although the boundaries between these two modes of care are not as sharply defined in practice as the theoretical distinction suggests, the contrast remains analytically valuable. It sheds light on the way care is conceptualized within our society and reflects the gendered structure of care work and responsibility. "Caring for" involves responding to the concrete, particular needs of others: physical, spiritual, intellectual, psychological and emotional. This care may be provided by oneself, by another individual or by a collective entity. Typical examples are as follows: I take care of myself; a mother cares for her child; a nurse cares for hospital patients; and the Red Cross provides care for victims of an earthquake. What unifies these examples is their shared foundation in the human condition: People have physical and psychological needs that require active engagement and response. These needs are, in part, shaped by social and cultural conditions, and they are addressed through various social practices that differ across societies ([12] pp. 173–4).

4.2.3 Living, Feeling and the Art of Self-Understanding Through Autobiography

We can live in a state of inertia, not as we wish to live, but merely by continuing as we began ([12] pp. 173–4). Yet this is not truly life; it is merely self-preservation extended over time. Life can be simply what happens to us, but it can also be more:

It can become the work of composing atoms of meaning through which we glimpse the desire for transcendence. We are entrusted with the task of discovering the art of living. Describing an affective lived experience involves a set of discursive operations: naming what we happen to feel, making explicit the underlying cognitive act and describing the expressive phenomenality of the emotion. One of the most comprehensive classical analyses of the practice of affective self-comprehension can be found in Aristotle's *Rhetoric*, in which emotional states are analytically examined [13]. Although Aristotle's primary intention was to provide a foundation for the art of rhetoric, and within that framework, to develop an understanding of emotional life that could support persuasive communication, his work holds profound implications for a phenomenology of affective experience. It emphasizes the need for self-examination as a means to understand both the origin and trajectory of our emotions. If we can grasp which mental disposition gives rise to a specific emotion, who typically experiences that emotional state and under what circumstances, we will possess essential, if not wholly sufficient, insights for gaining greater mastery over our modes of being [14].

Is autobiography a kind of medicine? A *sui generis* therapy? To address this question, we must return to antiquity, when the Greeks coined the imperative *epimelesthai heautou*, "take care of yourself", and the Romans later discovered that *otium* (withdrawal from public life) could act as both a remedy for the soul and a restorative for the body, *cura sui* in its fullest sense [2]. Autobiographical work can indeed exhibit analgesic effects. It may act through mechanisms such as dissolution, coexistence, recomposition, invention and depersonalization. These processes suggest that autobiographical writing is not only a narrative endeavour but also a therapeutic one. Demetrio argued that to truly understand who we are, we need memory, the faculty that constantly resists oblivion in the daily labour of self-formation [15]. This aligns with the insights of Jerome Bruner, who maintained that writing one's life story is not merely a matter of chronicling facts but rather a search for meaning and the very shape of the self: "One should, I believe, end an autobiography by trying to define what one means by oneself. And yet it is a desperate enterprise, for the moment one begins to think about it, it becomes clear that the boundaries of personality melt away like snow in the sun" ([16] p. 56). International scholars have reinforced this view. For Paul Ricœur, autobiography is the site of narrative identity, where the self is not revealed as a fixed substance but emerges through the ongoing act of employment, organizing events into a coherent story that reflects both constancy and transformation over time [17]. Georges Gusdorf suggested earlier that the act of writing one's own life is fundamentally pedagogical, a means of reaching towards self-knowledge and of integrating fragmented experience into a meaningful whole [18]. Autobiography is, therefore, not merely retrospective; it is prospective. It allows the individual to imagine possible selves and reconfigure the past in ways that foster healing, coherence and even ethical awareness. Sidonie Smith and Julia Watson argue that, "Life writing is performative—it does not just reflect a life but helps to shape and revise it" [19]. Autobiographical practice serves as a powerful tool for personal development in educational and therapeutic contexts alike. Whether framed as *cura sui*, narrative therapy or reflective writing, its power lies in the capacity to generate insight, enable reorientation and support the construction of a more coherent and liveable self.

4.3 The Ages of Life: From Early Childhood to Adulthood

Human development across the lifespan is a complex and dynamic process encompassing biological, psychological and social dimensions. Among the most influential theoretical frameworks for understanding identity formation and human relationships is Erik H. Erikson's theory of psychosocial development [20]. This model outlines eight distinct stages, each characterized by a specific developmental crisis (see Table 4.1). These stages are not isolated; instead, each provides the foundation for the next, making the resolution of psychosocial conflicts a cumulative process.

According to Erikson, the first stage spans from birth to approximately 18 months, during which the infant faces the crisis of trust versus mistrust. The quality of parental care plays a critical role in resolving this conflict positively. At this stage, John Bowlby's attachment theory becomes relevant [21], positing that the bond between the child and caregiver is a biologically programmed system aimed at ensuring protection and affective development. Secure attachment enables the child to explore the environment, regulate emotions and develop positive expectations about future relationships. Bowlby emphasized that inconsistent or neglectful caregiving can lead to dysfunctional internal working models. Subsequently, Mary Salter Ainsworth formalized three primary attachment styles (secure, insecure-avoidant and insecure-ambivalent) through experimental observation in the "Strange Situation" paradigm [22]. Secure attachment has been

Table 4.1 Erik H. Erikson's theory of psychosocial development

Stag	Age	Psychosocial conflict	Positive outcome	Negative outcome
1	0–1 year	Trust vs. mistrust	Trust in caregivers and the world	Fear and mistrust
2	1–3 years	Autonomy vs. shame/doubt	Independence and self-control	Dependency and shame
3	3–6 years	Initiative vs. guilt	Initiative and decision-making	Guilt and inhibition
4	6–12 years	Industry vs. inferiority	Competence and productivity	Feelings of inferiority
5	12–18 years	Identity vs. role confusion	Stable self-identity	Confusion about self
6	18–35 years	Intimacy vs. isolation	Deep relationships	Emotional isolation
7	35–65 years	Generativity vs. stagnation	Care and productivity	Self-absorption and stagnation
8	65+ years	Integrity vs. despair	Wisdom and acceptance	Regret and despair

associated with enhanced emotional regulation, empathy and relational autonomy during preschool and school age. Conversely, its absence may predispose individuals to social difficulties, mood disorders and identity-related issues, with long-term implications extending into adulthood.

During adolescence (12–18 years), individuals encounter the developmental crisis of identity versus role confusion. Adolescents strive to understand their place in the world by aligning their internal self-concept with external expectations. This stage involves a redefinition of family relationships, exploration of social identity and processing of bodily changes. Neuroscientific studies have confirmed that adolescence is a period of profound brain restructuring. Daniel J. Siegel describes the adolescent brain as undergoing "remodelling", marked by intense synaptic reorganization, which renders individuals emotionally vulnerable but also creatively potent [23]. Laurence Steinberg notes that the limbic system, responsible for emotional reactivity, matures earlier than the prefrontal cortex, which governs inhibitory control and planning, leading to a neuro-emotional imbalance that explains typical adolescent impulsivity [24]. Jeffrey Arnett introduced the concept of emerging adulthood to characterize the 18–25 age range as a distinct phase, marked by instability in housing, employment and relationships, extending the identity exploration process [25]. This notion is particularly pertinent in post-industrial societies, where transitions to adulthood are increasingly diverse. Entering adulthood (from approximately age 30 onwards), individuals face the dialectic of generativity versus stagnation. The task here is to balance personal fulfilment with contributing to others, through parenting, work or volunteering. Failure to achieve this balance may lead to narcissism, isolation and existential emptiness.

Individuals confront the final psychosocial crisis in late adulthood: ego integrity versus despair. Those who have constructed a coherent life narrative may achieve a sense of wisdom, accepting loss and facing physical decline with equanimity. Conversely, a sense of failure may lead to despair and fear of death. A critical concern in aging is the risk of social isolation, often exacerbated by bereavement, retirement, geographic dispersion of family and chronic illness. Julianne Holt-Lunstad and colleagues' meta-analyses have demonstrated that social isolation poses a greater mortality risk than smoking or obesity [26]. It is also associated with increased rates of depression and cognitive decline. Interventions such as intergenerational support networks, cohousing and promotion of active volunteering among the elderly have proven effective in mitigating these risks and fostering positive aging. Erikson himself reflected on the interplay between the first and last stages of life, and the notion that unresolved stagnation can lead to depression:

> In the most vital cultures, children mature mentally in a unique way through their interaction with older people. [...] The changes induced by time – such as increased life expectancy – require new and profound re-ritualizations capable of ensuring more meaningful exchanges between the beginning and the end of life, a more defined synthesis of stages, and possibly a more active and anticipatory participation in the face of death. For all these things, I believe the appropriate word will be wisdom, just as it will be despair. [...] The absence of this new involvement seems to be the nostalgic theme

> underlying the manifest symptoms that drive older individuals to seek psychotherapy. The most frequent reason for their despair is, in fact, a recurring and prolonged sense of stagnation. ([20] p. 61)

Institutionalization in long-term care facilities also warrants reflection. Many elderly individuals spend their final years in nursing homes and have the right not only to competent care—like all people—but also to relationships with professionals who understand their experience of marginalization and loneliness. It is essential in the healthcare field to recognize that individuals seeking help from nurses, physicians and pharmacists carry life stage-specific experiences. As described by Maila Mislej [27], the nursing profession underwent a significant transformation in the 1970s, driven by the New Nursing movement in Anglo-Saxon countries, redefining the nurse's role in holistic care. By contrast, Denmark and Sweden have implemented ambitious aging policies. These countries have repurposed traditional nursing homes into senior-dedicated apartments, socialization spaces, multi-age day centres and programmes promoting healthy aging. In these supportive housing units, if an older person presses a button, a caregiver promptly responds in person—rather than through a phone call. Home care services are so widespread that 20% of the elderly population receives 24-h assistance year-round.

4.4 Aesthetics and Cosmetics: Beauty Will Save the World

Beauty, understood not merely as an aesthetic attribute but as a subjective perception of harmony and well-being, plays a significant role in an individual's quality of life. Taking care of one's body, through daily practices of hygiene, cosmetics and personal wellness, represents not only an expression of self-esteem but also a fundamental tool for maintaining a psychophysical balance. In this context, cosmetics serve a function that goes far beyond the surface: They contribute to the reinforcement of personal identity, the management of body image and, in many cases, the restoration of a sense of dignity, particularly in the presence of debilitating illnesses. The use of cosmetics has ancient origins, rooted in the earliest human civilizations. Egyptians, Greeks, Romans, Mesopotamians and many other cultures developed rudimentary tools and artisanal preparations to beautify the body, protect the skin and perform religious or social rituals. Ointments, natural pigments, aromatic oils and coloured powders were employed not only for decorative purposes but also with symbolic, spiritual and protective meanings. This long-standing tradition demonstrates that care for physical appearance has been perceived, in every era, as an integral part of both individual and collective identity, revealing a cultural continuity that persists to this day. Aesthetic care is not the exclusive domain of any one gender. Both men and women benefit equally from the conscious use of cosmetic products. Cultural and social shifts have fostered a growing male interest in physical appearance in recent decades, leading to an increasingly inclusive cosmetics market. This evolution demands that healthcare professionals, particularly pharmacists working in private community pharmacies, possess up-to-date and comprehensive knowledge of not only active ingredients and formulations but also the empathetic and communicative dimensions of cosmetic counselling. In clinical contexts, the importance of beauty becomes even more pronounced when dealing with chronic or oncological illnesses. Disease, in addition to compromising organic health, often deeply affects a patient's self-image. Invasive treatments, such as chemotherapy or radiotherapy, can lead to visible side effects, including hair loss, skin alterations or weight fluctuations, that have a negative impact on self-perception. In such circumstances, the pharmacist has both the opportunity and the responsibility to intervene with sensitivity and expertise, offering targeted cosmetic solutions aimed at restoring the patient's sense of control over their body and promoting a lived experience of beauty despite the illness. In conclusion, beauty and body care are not secondary aspects of human life but are deeply interconnected with health, psychological well-being and social relationships. The pharmacist, as a healthcare professional, is called upon to recognize and enhance this dimension, contributing through thoughtful cosmetic advice to the construction of an integrated care pathway that respects the person in their entirety. Even in the Greek world during the time of Aristotle, beauty was associated with spaces and moments that were not necessarily utilitarian or essential but which, like philosophy itself, were savoured and experienced for the pure pleasure of the individual. Beauty, in this context, was not merely a functional concept but one tied to the intellectual and sensory enjoyment of life. At the same time, a life devoted to the polis, civic engagement and public action also gave rise to achievements imbued with beauty, which individuals would then contemplate as expressions of collective and aesthetic excellence.

James Hillman, the influential Jungian psychologist and founder of archetypal psychology, regarded beauty not as a mere aesthetic luxury but as a fundamental necessity for the soul [27]. Critiquing modernity's fixation on utility and efficiency, he warned that the suppression of beauty leads to a disenchanted, psychologically impoverished world. Drawing from Neoplatonic tradition, Hillman revived the idea of *anima mundi*, the soul of the world, proposing that beauty is an objective, animating presence in reality, not just a subjective impression. His reinterpretation of Fyodor Dostoyevsky's dictum, "Beauty will save the world" [28] shifted the emphasis from moral idealism to psychological immediacy: Beauty, for Hillman, is not a didactic solution but a presence that calls us into a deeper, more vital relationship with life. This principle extended to his clinical work, where he advocated for beauty as a therapeutic force, whether through art, poetry, myth or the intentional design of healing spaces. His essays and lectures on a "politics of beauty" argued for its reintegration into civic life, challenging the stark functionalism of urban and institutional environments.

This vision finds tangible expression in hospitals like Zurich's Children's Hospital [29], with its restorative gardens and light-filled spaces, or Barcelona's Sant Pau Modernist Site [30], where architecture itself becomes a conduit for healing. For Hillman, beauty was neither frivolous nor passive. It was an active encounter with the sacred, essential to mending the fragmented modern psyche.

4.5 Psychotropic Drugs, Illegal Drugs and Drug Addiction

> While heading to the library, I encountered Bill. This evening he is taking me out. I can hardly contain my excitement at the thought of what might unfold. I feel as though I am embarking on an entirely new journey—one that opens unimaginable doors. I feel like Alice in Wonderland. Perhaps Lewis Carroll himself experimented with drugs.
>
> Dear, warm, intimate diary,
>
> What an incredible, enlightening, and exhilarating week this has been! Truly, it has been uhuuh! the most extraordinary experience of my life. Do you recall I mentioned I had a date with Bill? On Friday, he introduced me to a type of amphetamine, and on Saturday, a different one. Taking them felt like riding a blazing star through the Milky Way no, a million, a trillion times better.
>
> Initially, I was somewhat apprehensive, as Bill had to inject the substance into my arm. I remembered how much I used to fear injections when I was hospitalized, but this was different. Now I am eager to try them again. Truly. It is no surprise they are colloquially called "rockets". I could barely control myself – in fact, I could not have even if I had wanted to, and I did not want to. I danced in ways I never imagined possible for someone as shy and introverted as myself. I felt powerful, liberated, at ease—a new, improved specimen of a different and superior species. What madness! What a marvel! Truly. ([31] p. 50)

What is a drug? What is a drug user? The figure of the drug user in common discourse is frequently associated with the world of hippies, social unrest and nonconformity to established norms. Similarly, drug dealers are often conflated with users and addicts, and those involved in illicit trafficking. This simplification extends further, with distinctions between 'hard' drugs (such as heroin and cocaine) and "soft" drugs (such as cannabis) often blurred. Moreover, there is a prevalent belief that the use of a single joint inevitably leads to heroin injection. Such misconceptions are perpetuated by an extensive media landscape, including films, documentaries and, more recently, a proliferation of popular television series on the subject.

This paragraph does not aim to exhaustively reconstruct the motivations of individuals who begin using drugs, nor the journeys of those who manage to recover from addiction. However, it is essential to reflect on the importance of healthcare professionals—including pharmacists—being adequately prepared to engage with individuals who use psychoactive substances. Throughout their careers, pharmacists may encounter patients undergoing rehabilitation and detoxification processes.

According to the WHO, the use of psychoactive substances constitutes one of the foremost global public health challenges, with profound individual, familial and societal impacts. The 2024 World Drug Report, published by the United Nations Office on Drugs and Crime, estimates that approximately 292 million people worldwide, around 5.6% of the global population aged 15–64, have used a psychoactive substance at least once in the previous year [32]. Substance use patterns vary significantly across gender and age groups. Data indicates that men represent about 70% of all drug users, while women account for the remaining 30%. However, women tend to be more vulnerable to the health and social consequences of drug use, including stigmatization and limited access to treatment services [33]. In terms of age demographics, substance use is most prevalent among young adults, with peak usage observed in the 18–25 age group, which displays significantly higher rates than other age categories. There has also been a rise in drug use among adolescents aged 15–17 in recent years, often facilitated by easier access through digital platforms and the normalization of cannabis consumption in certain geographic areas [34].

In today's globalized context, we are witnessing an acceleration of social and productive dynamics that demand an almost totalizing standard of individual performance. Individuals are expected to perform multiple tasks in increasingly limited time frames, maintaining high levels of efficiency and perfection. This phenomenon, characteristic of a deregulated and technocratic capitalism, has generated a widespread climate of stress and anxiety, accompanied by a marked increase in the consumption of psychotropic medications and psychoactive substances [35]. The constant pressure for self-optimization and rapid adaptation leads not only to psychological fatigue but also to a deep identity crisis. Philosopher Günther Anders, in his concept of "Promethean shame", has already highlighted this condition: faced with his own technological creations, modern man perceives himself as inadequate, inferior to the very machines he has produced [36]. In this logic, human subjectivity becomes a device to be optimized, rendered productive and competitive through continuous self-monitoring and self-correction. The globalized individual no longer compares themselves to others, but to an abstract, unattainable standard, thereby internalizing the logic of performance as the dominant mode of existence. Within this framework, psychoactive substances assume an increasingly central role. They are no longer used solely for recreational purposes or escapism, but rather as tools for social adaptation. Far from being mere accessories to leisure, they become instruments for mood regulation, productivity enhancement and social integration, reshaping the self in alignment with external expectations [37]. Subjectivity is no longer inherent, but chemically produced, in what might be described as a system of pharmacological biopolitics. This scenario outlines a future in which psychoactive substance use may become indispensable for social and economic participation. Byung-Chul Han observes that the performance-oriented society produces individuals who self-exploit in the name of freedom, engaging in a form of neuronal violence that finds in psychotropic drugs a means of normalization [38]. Confronted with the imperative to remain constantly efficient, joyful and competitive, chemistry becomes the new ally of neoliberal governance. The risk is the erosion of authentic subjectivity, replaced by an adaptive personality tailored to the demands of the global market. In light of this complex landscape, it is imperative that all healthcare professionals, including pharmacists, develop specific competencies in the management, support and communication with individuals who use psychoactive substances. This responsibility is not only clinical but also ethical and social, especially considering that pharmacists may be among the few healthcare providers with regular contact with such individuals during their rehabilitation journeys. Therefore, it is crucial to promote a non-judgemental, empathetic approach, grounded in active listening and collaboration with other healthcare professionals.

4.6 Pharmacist's Burnout

Burnout, defined by the WHO as a syndrome resulting from chronic workplace stress that has not been successfully managed, is an increasingly widespread phenomenon among healthcare professionals. Physicians, nurses, pharmacists and other care providers are routinely exposed to high emotional and operational demands, exacerbated by long shifts, life-critical responsibilities and institutional pressure. The data are particularly concerning among physicians. A 2022 survey by the Mayo Clinic, published in Mayo Clinic Proceedings, found that 63% of physicians in the United States reported symptoms of burnout, an alarming increase from 44% in 2017 [39]. Similar studies in Europe indicate a prevalence ranging from 30% to 50%, depending on the speciality and working conditions [40]. A multicentre study conducted across 12 European countries, for example, reported that 43% of physicians surveyed exhibited at least one significant symptom of burnout, with higher rates in countries experiencing severe staffing shortages [41]. The problem is equally widespread among nurses and allied health professionals. A 2021 European survey involving over 2000 healthcare workers in Germany, Belgium and the Netherlands showed that more than 50% reported high levels of emotional exhaustion and job-related stress [42]. The COVID-19 pandemic has further exacerbated this situation, increasing the workload and emotional burden of frontline workers across the continent. Pharmacists, although often overlooked in such analyses, are not immune to burnout. Hospital pharmacists and those working in community or primary care settings frequently report high levels of occupational stress and exhaustion. An international study published in 2020 revealed that around 40% of pharmacists experienced burnout symptoms, largely due to workload, role ambiguity and lack of organizational support [43]. The consequences of burnout are serious for not only the individuals affected, who face increased risks of depression, substance misuse and suicide, but also the quality of patient care. Evidence shows that higher burnout levels are associated with more frequent clinical errors, reduced patient communication and increased workforce turnover [44].

A paradigm shift is urgently needed. Burnout should not be viewed as a personal weakness but as a systemic issue that demands structural solutions. Effective strategies include the promotion of organizational well-being, emotional resilience training, improved leadership practices and the development of more humane and sustainable work environments.

4.7 Practice Time

1. What do you mean by the concept of self-care?
2. What are some of the most common interpretations of this concept?
3. What does the myth of Cronos tell us, and why is it important?
4. What is burnout?

5. According to data reported in the chapter, are more men or women addicted to drugs? In your opinion, why is this so?
6. What is the sense of aesthetics and cosmetics for a person with a disease?

References

1. Plato. Apology of Socrates. In: Cooper JM, editor. Plato: complete works. Indianapolis: Hackett Publishing; 1997.
2. Foucault M. Le souci de soi [The care of the self]. Paris: Gallimard; 1984.
3. Seneca. Epistulae Morales ad Lucilium. Letter 66. In: Moral letters to Lucilius. Gummere RM, translator. Cambridge: Harvard University Press; 1917.
4. Arendt H. The human condition. Chicago: University of Chicago Press; 1958.
5. Levinas E. Totalité et infini: essai sur l'extériorité. Paris: Livre de Poche; 1991.
6. Stein E. L'essere finito e l'essere eterno. Rone: Città Nuova; 1991.
7. Epicurus. Lettera a Meneceo. In: Opere. Turin: Einaudi; 1970.
8. Aristotle. Nicomachean ethics. Book I, 1094a. In: Barnes J, editor. The complete works of Aristotle. Princeton: Princeton University Press; 1984.
9. Zambrano M. Persona y democracia: una historia sacrificial. Madrid: Siruela; 1989.
10. Heidegger M. Sein und Zeit [Being and time]. Tübingen: Niemeyer; 1927.
11. Nussbaum MC. The therapy of desire: theory and practice in Hellenistic ethics. Princeton: Princeton University Press; 1996.
12. Tronto JC. Women and caring: what can feminists learn about morality from caring? In: Jaggar AM, Bordo SR, editors. Gender/body/knowledge: feminist reconstructions of being and knowing. New Brunswick: Rutgers University Press; 1989. p. 172–87.
13. Aristotle. Rhetoric. Book II, 1378a. In: Barnes J, editor. The complete works of Aristotle. Princeton: Princeton University Press; 1984.
14. Mortari L. The wisdom of the heart: thinking, emotions, feeling thoughts. Bucharest: Zeta Books; 2023.
15. Demetrio D. Raccontarsi. In: L'autobiografia come cura di sé. Milano: Raffaello Cortina; 1996.
16. Bruner J. In search of mind: essays in autobiography. New York: Harper & Row; 1983.
17. Ricœur P. Oneself as another. University of Chicago Press; 1992.
18. Gusdorf G. Conditions and limits of autobiography. In: Olney J, editor. Autobiography: essays theoretical and critical. Princeton: Princeton University Press; 1980. p. 28–48.
19. Smith S, Watson J. Reading autobiography: a guide for interpreting life narratives. Minneapolis: University of Minnesota Press; 2010.
20. Erikson EH. The life cycle completed: a review. London: Norton & Company; 1982.
21. Bowlby J. Attachment and loss, vol. 1. Attachment. New York: Basic Books; 1969.
22. Salter Ainsworth MD, Blehar MC, Waters E, Wall SN. Patterns of attachment. A psychological study of the strange situation. London, New York: Psychology Press; 2015.
23. Siegel DJ. Brainstorm: the power and purpose of the teenage brain. New York: TarcherPerigee; 2013.
24. Steinberg L. Age of opportunity: lessons from the new science of adolescence. Boston: Houghton Mifflin Harcourt; 2014.
25. Arnett JJ. Emerging adulthood: a theory of development from the late teens through the twenties. Am Psychol. 2000;55(5):469–80.
26. Holt-Lunstad J, Smith TB, Layton JB. Social relationships and mortality risk: a meta-analytic review. PLoS Med. 2010;7(7):e1000316.
27. Hillman J. The thought of the heart and the soul of the world. Thompson: Spring Publications; 1981.
28. Dostoyevsky F. The idiot. Garnett C, translator. New York: Macmillan; 1913.

29. Zürich's Childrens Hospital. Internet. Available from: https://www.kispi.uzh.ch/en.
30. Sant Pau Hospital Modernist Site, Barcelona. Available from: https://www.spain.info/en/places-of-interest/sant-pau-modernist-site/.
31. Anonymous. Go ask Alice. Upper Saddle River: Prentice Hall; 1971.
32. United Nations Office on Drugs and Crime (UNODC). World drug report 2024. Vienna: UNODC; 2024. Available from: https://www.unodc.org/unodc/en/data-and-analysis/wdr2024.html.
33. World Health Organization. Health and social responses to drug problems: a European guide. Geneva: WHO; 2022.
34. European Monitoring Centre for Drugs and Drug Addiction (EMCDDA). European Drug Report 2024: trends and developments. Luxembourg: Publications Office of the European Union. p. 2024.
35. Ehrenberg A. The weariness of the self: diagnosing the history of depression in the contemporary age. Montréal: McGill-Queen's University Press; 2016.
36. Anders G. Die Antiquiertheit des Menschen. Zurich: Arche; 1961.
37. Rose N. Governing the soul: the shaping of the private self. Stanmore: Free Association Books; 1990.
38. Han B-C. The burnout society. Redwood City: Stanford Briefs; 2015.
39. Shanafelt TD, West CP, Dyrbye LN, Trockel M, Tutty M, Wang H, Carlasare LE, Sinsky C. Changes in burnout and satisfaction with work-life integration in physicians during the first 2 years of the COVID-19 pandemic. Mayo Clin Proc. 2022;97(12):2248–58.
40. Rotenstein LS, Torre M, Ramos MA, Rosales RC, Guille C, Sen S, Mata DA. Prevalence of burnout among physicians: a systematic review. JAMA. 2018;320(11):1131–40.
41. Domagała A, Klich J, Dubas-Jakóbczyk K, Orlik M, Szetela B, Kaczmarczyk M, et al. Burnout among healthcare professionals in Europe: a systematic review and meta-analysis. Int J Occup Med Environ Health. 2022;35(3):265–86.
42. Van Gerven E, De Witte H, Sermeus W, Euwema M. Linking communication skills and burnout among healthcare professionals: a systematic review. Patient Educ Couns. 2021;104(4):805–16.
43. Johnson SJ, O'Connor EM, Jacobs S, Hassell K, Ashcroft DM. The relationships among work stress, strain and self-reported errors in UK community pharmacy. Res Social Adm Pharm. 2020;16(1):96–106.
44. Dyrbye LN, West CP, Sinsky CA, Goeders LE, Satele DV, Shanafelt TD. Medical licensure questions and physician reluctance to seek care for mental health conditions. Mayo Clin Proc. 2017;92(10):1486–93.

Chapter 5
The Italian Case Study

5.1 Introduction

In the context of the ongoing reorganization of territorial healthcare following the COVID-19 pandemic, Italian pharmacies have emerged as key players in strengthening the National Health Service (SSN), particularly in the management of chronic diseases and the provision of community-based services. Their widespread presence across the country and the strong trust they enjoy among citizens position them as indispensable points of care, ensuring equitable access to essential health services. Pharmacies increasingly offer not only medicinal products but also a wide range of healthcare services, including health screenings and telemedicine, thereby contributing to prevention and the monitoring of public health. The 2024 Budget Law introduced a new remuneration model aimed at enhancing the financial sustainability of pharmacies, especially those with a lower turnover, and promoting the transfer of medicines from direct distribution by local health authorities to conventional distribution channels. This reform seeks to improve therapeutic adherence, particularly among chronic patients, by facilitating easier access to medicines through a professional and capillary network. In this context, the experimental programme known as the "Service Pharmacy" has been extended through 2024. The social and healthcare role of pharmacies has also been formally recognized by the Constitutional Court, which emphasized their contribution to the protection of public health. Pharmacies served as essential reference points for the population during the COVID-19 emergency, ensuring safe access to medicines and supporting diagnostic testing and vaccination campaigns. The sustainability of the pharmacy system is supported by a balance between its healthcare mission and commercial activity, which enables continued operation even in peripheral or underserved areas. Pharmacies recorded approximately 720 million visits in 2023, averaging 3000 visits per month per pharmacy. The presence of 1800 night-time pharmacies and over 7200 rural pharmacies, many of which receive public subsidies, underscores the

S. Leoncini, *The Relationship between Pharmacists and Patients*, New Paradigms in Healthcare, https://doi.org/10.1007/978-3-032-21249-8_5

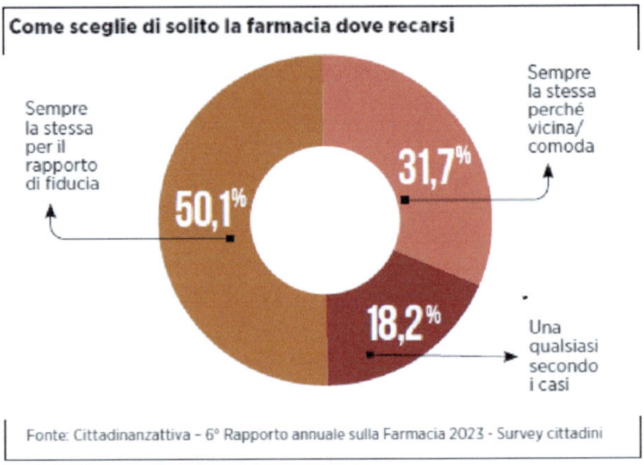

Fig. 5.1 Federfarma Italian Pharmacies 2024. (Printed in April 2024)

sector's commitment to providing continuous service, including in low-density areas. Data also show a growing demand for health services: blood pressure monitoring, prescription reservation and home delivery are among the most requested, reflecting the needs of an aging population with increasing chronic conditions. A concrete example of pharmacies' commitment to preventive healthcare is the "Cuore di Donna in Farmacia" campaign, conducted in three Italian regions, which identified a significant proportion of women at high cardiovascular risk, including asymptomatic individuals. Similarly, the expansion of telemedicine services, with nearly half a million services delivered in 2023, has represented a strategic innovation, improving both the access to and timeliness of care. Future projections indicate a strengthening of the role of pharmacies as central hubs for community-based care, in close collaboration with the SSN. The integration of digital services, the provision of health screenings, ongoing professional training and cooperation with organizations such as Federfarma and Cittadinanzattiva lay the foundation for a more inclusive, efficient and patient-centred healthcare model. In this evolving scenario, Italian pharmacies reaffirm their role not only as healthcare providers but also as key social factors contributing to the resilience and sustainability of the national health system (Fig. 5.1).

5.2 Pharmacies in Rural Places

More than 7200 rural pharmacies operate in municipalities or towns in Italy with fewer than 5000 inhabitants, collectively serving a population of over 10 million people. This means that approximately one-third of all Italian pharmacies are located in small communities. Among these, 4400 are classified as "subsidized rural pharmacies", situated in areas with fewer than 3000 residents. These facilities alone provide essential pharmaceutical and health-related services to more than 5 million individuals. Notably, 2000 of these pharmacies are located in very small towns with fewer than 1500 inhabitants, and serve nearly 2 million people, many of whom are elderly and have limited mobility. Rural pharmacies are more than mere dispensaries of medicines; they are indispensable health outposts in geographically and socially disadvantaged areas. They often represent the only easily accessible point of care, particularly in remote mountain villages, small islands or coastal hamlets far from urban centres. Their presence ensures a continuous and reliable link between citizens and the healthcare system for 24 hours a day, 365 days a year. Because of their unique and critical function, rural pharmacies receive financial support from regional governments. This support varies across regions, depending on local legislative frameworks, and is aimed at ensuring the economic sustainability of pharmacies operating in contexts with limited population density and reduced commercial viability. The year 2024 represents a pivotal moment for rural pharmacies in Italy, as a number of policy and financial measures came into effect that will significantly influence their operations. Chief among these is the transition to a new remuneration system for medicines dispensed under agreement with the SSN. Effective as of 1 March 2024, this model introduces a hybrid reimbursement structure: 25% of the pharmacy's margin is calculated as a percentage of the drug's price (6%), while the remaining 75% is provided through fixed quotas. Additional "typological" quotas are allocated to pharmacies that previously benefited from SSN discount exemptions, such as full exemptions, flat-rate discounts of 1.5% or reductions of 60%, thereby channelling more resources towards the most vulnerable pharmacies. This change not only reinforces their financial viability but also recognizes the professional value of their healthcare role. A central aim of the new remuneration scheme is to make it more cost-effective for the SSN to transfer drugs from direct distribution by local health units to the more accessible conventional distribution network offered by pharmacies. This is particularly advantageous for residents of remote areas, who often face significant logistical challenges in obtaining medications. At the same time, the reform bolsters the sustainability of rural and small-scale pharmacies, ensuring that even Italy's most isolated communities continue to receive equitable healthcare access. Another major development in 2024 relates to Italy's National Recovery and Resilience Plan, specifically under Mission 5: Territorial Cohesion. This initiative includes targeted investments to enhance rural pharmacy services in municipalities with fewer than 3000 inhabitants. As part of a public call launched in late 2021, funds have been allocated to support structural improvements in these pharmacies, enabling them to expand their range of services, improve chronic patient care and implement telemedicine technologies. A second funding call is expected to be issued within 2024, aimed at co-financing the purchase of equipment and services that will further elevate the role of rural pharmacies as frontline healthcare providers. These developments, namely, the revised remuneration system and National Recovery and Resilience Plan investments, reflect the growing recognition by the Italian government and parliament of rural pharmacies as vital pillars of local healthcare infrastructure. They are not only essential for reducing territorial disparities in healthcare access but also demonstrate a model of adaptability and commitment on the part of pharmacists themselves. These professionals continue to invest both economically and professionally to meet the evolving needs of their communities that, while often perceived as marginal, are in fact central to the country's cultural and geographic identity. Various solidarity initiatives have been implemented within the pharmacy sector itself to further support rural and low-income pharmacies. Federfarma, the national association representing pharmacy owners, has established an internal solidarity fund to assist pharmacies with low revenue. Hundreds of such pharmacies received financial support through this mechanism from 2014 to 2022, an intervention that proved especially crucial during the most challenging economic phases. The number of pharmacies requiring such assistance has steadily declined over the years, thanks, in part, to governmental policies that reduced or eliminated mandatory SSN discounts for low-turnover pharmacies. In addition, the National Social Security and Assistance Institution for Pharmacists has introduced specific grants for rural pharmacists with limited income. Although temporarily suspended during the COVID-19 pandemic to reallocate resources for emergency support, the grant was reinstated in 2022 and continues to provide critical aid to those operating under financial strain. In conclusion, rural and small pharmacies in Italy represent far more than just points of pharmaceutical access. They are essential community institutions, helping to preserve the health and well-being of populations often neglected by mainstream healthcare infrastructure. Their continued support through public investment, regulatory reform and professional solidarity will be key to ensuring a more inclusive and territorially cohesive healthcare system in the years to come.

5.3 Reform of the Pharmacy Degree Course

The reform of the master's degree in pharmacy, introduced by Interministerial Decree No. 651 of 5 July 2022 [1], established a directly qualifying educational path for the pharmacy profession, eliminating the need for a separate state examination. The decree, implementing Articles 1 and 3 of Law No. 163 of 8 November 2021, stipulates that the single-cycle master's degree in pharmacy (Class LM-13) automatically grants professional qualification, provided the curriculum meets ministerial requirements. Specifically, the programme requires at least 300 European Credit Transfer and Accumulation System (ECTS) credits, balanced between theoretical courses, laboratory activities and mandatory internships in community pharmacies, hospitals or industrial settings. This approach ensures more uniform and professional training, aligning with European standards and reducing disparities among universities. Regarding specialization in hospital pharmacy, the programme spans four years, with the acquisition of 240 ECTS credits, of which at least 168 (70%) are reserved for professionalizing activities, practical training and internships. Each professionalizing ECTS credit corresponds to 30 hours of work, totalling a minimum of 5040 internship hours (approximately 1260 hours per year, with flexibility between 960 and 1500 hours, depending on the division between lectures and practical activities). Trainees must undergo annual rotations across different settings, with placements determined by availability. The internship in hospital pharmacy departments aims to provide trainees with comprehensive knowledge regarding the proper management of medications and medical devices within hospital settings. This includes developing competencies in generating consumption reports, conducting data analyses and performing monitoring activities (pharmacovigilance and medical device vigilance). Trainees will gain practical experience in procurement procedures through specialized tenders (technical specifications), participate in ward inspections and contribute to the management of the Therapeutic Formulary and Medical Device Registry. The internship in hospital Galenic laboratories is designed to equip trainees with specialized knowledge in the preparation of both sterile and non-sterile pharmaceutical formulations (magistral and officinal preparations), including parenteral nutrition bags and antineoplastic drugs. The programme emphasizes quality control procedures and provides training in clinical trials, including the evaluation of experimental protocols, management of investigational medicinal products and participation in ethical committee activities. The community pharmacy internship focuses on developing competencies in direct medication dispensing, monitoring and analysing general practitioners' prescription patterns and participating in inspection activities related to community pharmacies. Trainees will engage in prescription appropriateness control, contribute to administrative procedures concerning pharmacy licensing and wholesale drug distribution, and participate in technical control activities related to prosthetic care, supplementary healthcare services and integrated home care assistance. Assessment often involves presentations (PDF/PowerPoint) on topics agreed with supervisors, while attendance at lectures is mandatory. This pathway ensures comprehensive specialist training, preparing hospital pharmacists to work in complex, multidisciplinary healthcare environments.

5.4 Interviews with Experts: Interviews with a Psychologist in an Oncology Department in a Hospital; Daniela Scala and Titti Faggiano from SIFO

5.4.1 Interview with a Psychologist Working in an Oncology Department[1]

– What was your role in the oncology department, specifically in immunotherapy?

I worked as a clinical psychologist supporting adult cancer patients and their families. My work was structured and based on psychological screenings, as recommended by official guidelines. Some patients received ongoing support, while others were followed depending on their clinical condition: some weekly, others monthly. I was also involved during the highly delicate moment of diagnosis disclosure, following specific protocols

[1] No specific references have been made to the department or the hospital in order to respect the privacy of the patients, the psychologist and their colleagues. The interview was conducted on 10 March 2025.

for that phase. I used validated tools, such as the Distress Thermometer, developed by the National Comprehensive Cancer Network,[2] as well as the distress screening suggested by the Italian Society of Psycho-Oncology,[3] to assess psychological distress. The term 'distress' refers to a mix of emotional difficulties such as fatigue, anxiety, sadness and worry, that can significantly impact a patient's quality of life. The Distress Thermometer is effective because it captures this multidimensional experience.

– Do you believe psychological assessment and personalized care plans are useful for patients?

Absolutely. In my experience as a cognitive-behavioural therapist, I've seen first-hand the benefits of personalized approaches. Studies involving breast and lung cancer patients show that psychological support can significantly reduce anxiety and depression, measured using tools like the HADS (Hospital Anxiety and Depression Scale) [2]. Tailored interventions also improve treatment compliance. Patients are more likely to follow therapies consciously and consistently. This leads to lifestyle choices that better align with ongoing treatments.

– Do you see a connection between your work and narrative medicine?

Yes, there's a deep connection. When patients talk about their experience, especially during diagnosis, they begin reconstructing their own story. At first, trauma makes everything feel fragmented and chaotic. But through storytelling, even informal ones shared with friends or family, patients start making sense of what's happening. Over time, those fragments come together into a more coherent narrative. Occasionally, physicians and psychologists would deliver the diagnosis together, but unfortunately, that wasn't routine. It's crucial to give space to the patient's voice; narrative medicine starts there.

– How much impact does listening to the patient have on the healing process? Are there any scientific findings on this?

Listening plays a huge role. Medical students are required to take a psychology course, but in practice, not everyone chooses to collaborate with psychologists. However, when collaboration did happen, the outcomes were truly meaningful for both patients and the work environment. The oncology department is a very high-stress setting, and I was the only psychologist available. Guidelines on burn-out stress the importance of working as a team, not only for the well-being of healthcare providers but also for patients. When patients see a united, cohesive team, it boosts their trust and confidence. Healing is not just about treatments; it's also about human connection.

– Were there any words, episodes or events from this experience that particularly affected you?

Many moments were deeply moving. I learned so much from my patients, especially their ability to remain present. I remember one man who, despite his illness, lived fully in the moment, day by day, almost in a state of mindfulness. He remained present until the end and left a lasting impression. Another powerful experience involved working with ill parents who had young children. They often avoided talking about the illness with their kids, out of fear or the desire to protect them. But not knowing often causes more anxiety in children. Helping parents find the right words to communicate openly was one of the most delicate and meaningful aspects of my work.

– Do you think this type of service should be available in other healthcare settings, both in Italy and abroad?

Absolutely. I was fully dedicated to one department, but in many hospitals, psychologists are only brought in occasionally for specific consultations. This makes it difficult to

---

[2] Information about the Distress Thermometer is available on the National Comprehensive Cancer Network website in 71 languages. The English version is available from: https://www.nccn.org/docs/default-source/patient-resources/nccn_distress_thermometer.pdf?sfvrsn=ef1df1a2_10

[3] For further information, please visit https://www.ipos-society.org/federation/italy

provide consistent, long-term care even though some patients are followed for years. Unfortunately, funding for psycho-oncology is not always systematic. But this kind of support should be considered an integral part of treatment. Psychological care is not a luxury; it's a fundamental element of the healing process.

The interview with the psychologist working in an Italian oncology department of a hospital offers a compelling insight into the indispensable role of psychosocial support in cancer care. The integration of psychological screening tools, such as the Distress Thermometer and the guidelines from the Italian Society of Psycho-Oncology, which point to a structured, evidence-based approach to emotional care, is particularly striking. This not only aligns with best practices but also highlights the need for psychological assessments to be embedded within the broader therapeutic process. Psychological support, especially when provided alongside attentive physicians and pharmacists, significantly enhances the quality of care for oncology patients. The emotional burden in terminal or advanced stages of illness is often as profound as the physical one. The presence of a psychologist here can provide a crucial buffer, helping patients navigate fear, grief and existential distress. However, the interview reveals that even patients in earlier stages benefit greatly from having their emotional needs recognized and addressed. Personalized psychological interventions have been shown to reduce anxiety and depression, increase treatment adherence, and promote a sense of agency and dignity. The emphasis on narrative medicine, where the act of storytelling becomes therapeutic, is equally important. Encouraging patients to construct and reconstruct their own narratives allows for a reintegration of identity following the traumatic disruption of a cancer diagnosis. This process, when facilitated by clinicians who listen actively and compassionately, fosters a form of healing that extends beyond the physical. The interview also underscores the importance of interdisciplinary collaboration. When psychologists, physicians and pharmacists communicate and work together as a cohesive team, the patient perceives a unified front, an environment of trust and safety. This shared effort is especially crucial in high-stress environments such as oncology wards, where burnout is a real threat and continuity of care is paramount. In conclusion, the interview not only illuminates the essential role of the psychologist but also advocates for a holistic, team-based approach to care. Listening to patients, understanding their fears and offering tailored emotional support are not adjuncts to treatment; they are a fundamental component of healing for those in terminal phases and beyond.

5.4.2 *Interviews with Daniela Scala and Titti Faggiano from SIFO*[4]

5.4.2.1 Interview with Daniela Scala

– How long have you been working as a pharmacist, and what is your role within SIFO?

[4]The interviews were conducted on 22 July 2025.

- I have been working as a pharmacist since 1985, primarily in hospital pharmacy. I have been a member of SIFO for many years, holding various positions, including membership on the National Board and the Regional Secretariat. I currently coordinate the training area for healthcare professionals within the National Health Service and collaborate with other institutions to promote the pharmacist's role through continuous education. I also oversee thematic areas such as pharmacovigilance and scientific information. The latter is closely related to counselling, as it involves not only the dissemination of knowledge but also active listening to patients' needs. Over ten years ago, I completed a master's degree in narrative pharmacy, which was a turning point in my career. It enabled me to integrate clinical and chemical expertise with a more human, relational approach. I still coordinate a team composed mainly of young professionals and many pharmacy residents. I strongly believe in the value of dialogue with stakeholders and fostering meaningful professional relationships.
- What is the main mission of SIFO?
- SIFO works to enhance the role of hospital and healthcare service pharmacists through training, continuing education, research and professional networking. It also acts as a liaison with the national healthcare system and supports the ongoing improvement of pharmaceutical care quality.
- Do you see a connection between your work and narrative medicine?
- Absolutely. The pharmacist is often a liminal figure—visible yet not fully recognized—yet central to the care process. Narrative medicine has helped me appreciate the importance of listening, writing as a reparative tool and authentic encounters with patients. I have collaborated with SIMeN (Italian Society for Narrative Medicine) and continue to incorporate this approach into my daily practice.
- To what extent do you believe that listening to patients influences their healing process? Are there scientific studies supporting this?
- Patient listening is crucial. Counselling is not just about providing information; it's about understanding the patient's experience, daily challenges and fears. There is substantial scientific evidence, including studies on the placebo effect, that show how context and relational dynamics significantly impact treatment outcomes. Techniques such as teach-back, where patients are asked to repeat what they've understood, are validated tools that improve therapeutic adherence. There is also the concept of medication reconciliation: understanding what the patient actually takes, how they take it and what meaning they attribute to the therapy.
- Can you share any specific episodes from your professional experience that particularly struck you?
- I recall an engineer who initially refused to undergo clinical tests because he feared being mocked. He came to our centre very hesitant, and we welcomed him with understanding and respect for his fears. He would often call for reassurance. At one point, he told me, "I trust you, but I need you to tell me in person that there are no side effects". Another patient once said, "I come here because you care for the person, not just the disease. You don't make me feel guilty". These encounters remind me that treatment plans must be negotiated: for example, one patient explained that drinking a lot of water interfered with his work because of frequent restroom breaks. Others struggled with quitting smoking or reducing salt intake. All of this shows how essential it is to consider the patient's life context, not just the clinical guidelines.
- Do you believe that the recent reform making the pharmacy degree a qualifying title requires changes in how future pharmacists are trained, especially in terms of patient care?
- Yes, change is already underway. The notion of care is being increasingly discussed, not only as clinical treatment (cure), but as relational and human engagement (care). Future pharmacists need training not only in technical skills but also in communication, empa-

thy and relationship-building. The COVID-19 experience emphasized the importance of human contact: even a glance conveyed closeness and understanding.
- What does the word "care" mean to you, beyond its medical definition?
- It means being in service to others. Care has a deeply human and relational dimension. It is about presence, support and attention beyond the physical symptoms.
- What skills should a pharmacist have when beginning their professional career?
- They should possess basic competencies not only in pharmacology but also in communication, counselling and nonverbal language. Pharmacists need to be prepared to interact with people from diverse backgrounds, including those with disabilities or communication challenges, such as autistic patients. Listening is a multisensory act: it involves sound, visual perception and even interpreting silence. The hospital pharmacy specialization already includes a counselling module, and I believe similar training should be incorporated into community pharmacy education as well.
- What advice would you offer to future pharmacists to help them perform their role effectively?

Never forget that behind every prescription there is a human being. Train not only your technical knowledge but also your ability to relate. Learn to listen, observe and write. Have the courage to genuinely care.

5.4.2.2 Interview with Titti Faggiano

- How long have you been working as a pharmacist, and what is your role within SIFO?
- I have been working as a pharmacist for several decades, mainly in hospital pharmacy. I have been actively involved in SIFO for many years, covering various roles: regional secretary, scientific director and currently coordinator of training programmes within the National Health Service. I also lead the youth area and collaborate with various institutions to enhance the role of hospital pharmacists and promote a professional culture that combines technical and human competencies.
- What does SIFO do?
- SIFO represents over 3000 public-sector pharmacists out of approximately 4000 working in healthcare. The organization is structured into numerous technical-scientific areas that reflect the diverse specializations within the field. We work to promote the quality of pharmaceutical services through training, research, pharmacovigilance and innovation projects, many of which are led by younger colleagues. One of our current challenges is to build effective connections between the technical-scientific dimension and the often overlooked relational and communicative aspects of care.
- Do you see a connection between your work and narrative medicine?
- Absolutely. I completed a master's programme in narrative medicine with Dr. Marini and have since integrated this approach into my work at SIFO. We've promoted projects on "narrative pharmacovigilance" and patient listening. Narrative medicine teaches us that drugs are not just molecules, they often carry symbolic meaning for the patient, representing hope or safety. I try to honour this awareness in my daily practice: Hospital pharmacists often fill a relational void in the care pathway, acting not only as technical experts but also as human and social intermediaries. We interact with a wide range of stakeholders, physicians, nurses, administrators and suppliers, and we need effective communication tools and a mindset that goes beyond the community pharmacy model.
- To what extent do you believe listening to patients affects their healing? Is there scientific evidence to support this?
- Listening is essential and has a direct impact on treatment adherence and psychological well-being. There is robust evidence supporting this, including in the area of pharmacovigilance. Techniques such as teach-back, asking patients to repeat back what they've

understood, have proven to reduce errors and improve outcomes. In my experience, stepping out of one's comfort zone to embrace the complexity of each patient is crucial, especially in chronic or vulnerable situations where the pharmacist often becomes a trusted point of reference.

- Are there any episodes from your career that particularly left an impression on you?

Many. I remember a young woman in her early 30 s with a rare form of cancer. She was on pain management therapy, had lost her sense of taste and couldn't eat. She was also suffering from hallucinations caused by her medication. Working with clinical nutrition, we adapted her treatment to make it more palatable. She only had a week left to live, but that small gesture brought her relief. I also recall her father, who believed I could save his daughter; each phone call carried so much hope and unspoken grief. Another formative encounter was with a medical director who taught me the value of communication: He welcomed patients into his office and listened without judgement. I understood then that dialogue, not punishment, is the key to improving care pathways.

- What do you think about the recent reform that made the pharmacy degree automatically qualifying? Does this require changes in how future pharmacists are trained?
- Yes, it's an important turning point. The profession is evolving, and we now need training that includes relational and ethical dimensions, not just technical skills. The pandemic highlighted how essential contact, eye contact and human closeness are. We can no longer afford to train only technicians; we need people who are truly able to 'care'.
- What does the word care mean to you, beyond its medical definition?
- Care means time, listening and attention. It's also about reciprocity: being both caregiver and care receiver. It's the only way to prevent burnout and maintain balance. Care also defines the ethical and team climate we need among healthcare professionals. Without it, even the best technical skills are not enough.
- What tools should a pharmacist have at the start of their career?
- In addition to scientific knowledge, they need listening skills, interpersonal communication tools, an understanding of body language and basic training in counselling. It would be useful to include training in nonverbal communication, inclusion and interactions with neurodivergent patients, such as those on the autism spectrum. Pharmacists must be able to listen to what is not said, read context and adapt their communication to different needs.
- What advice would you give to young pharmacists to help them thrive in their profession?
- Never stop learning. Observe, listen, stay curious. Be open to innovation: Tools such as artificial intelligence can be useful, but they must not replace the human connection. The future of pharmacy lies in our ability to combine technological advancement with humanity.

5.4.2.3 A Reflection Based on the Interviews

In light of the interviews with Daniela Scala and Titti Faggiano, and in relation to recent qualitative studies conducted in the field of hospital pharmacy, a process of profound redefinition of the pharmacist's professional identity is emerging [3]. Articles that examine narrative pharmacy and group dynamics in hospital pharmacy [4] highlight how, beyond traditional technical and scientific expertise, there is a growing need for recognition and appreciation of the relational and narrative dimensions of the profession. It was observed in the first pilot study, conducted within the master's programme in pharmaceutical department management [5], that pharmacists perceive a certain sense of insecurity and lack of recognition within the national healthcare system. At the same time, however, they express a strong desire for autonomous growth and self-awareness through the use of narrative. The narratives collected, analysed using tools from narrative medicine and communication theory, emphasize the importance of respect, listening and human relationships in daily professional practice. Parallel to this, the study on teamwork in hospital pharmacy [6] revealed that the team is perceived primarily as a relationship rather than merely an organizational structure, with metaphors ranging from "a cog in a machine" to "a family." Nevertheless, significant challenges emerge in this context, such as a lack of leadership, absence of shared goals and the risk of burnout. Evidence exists which shows that counselling patients on medication and lifestyle modifications improves adherence, resulting in improved treatment outcomes, enhanced quality of life and better use of healthcare resources [7]. These findings resonate with the reflections of Scala and Faggiano, who, drawing on their experiences as hospital pharmacists and educators, emphasize that narrative pharmacy represents not only a more human and participatory method of care but also an important driver for professional training and development. Both recognize the introduction of communication, empathy and leadership skills as a necessary and urgent shift, especially in the context of the current reform of the qualifying pharmacy degree, which offers an opportunity to rethink educational content through a more humanistic lens. This leads to an emerging image of the pharmacist as no longer a mere dispenser of drugs but an integrated healthcare professional, capable of using narrative and relational skills as tools for improving care quality, fostering personal empowerment and strengthening their role within the healthcare system. There has been a growing interest in patients' subjective experiences, often explored through the narrative paradigm, within the social sciences applied to health, particularly in medical sociology and anthropology. The narration of illness, far from being a mere phenomenological description, represents a symbolic process through which individuals attempt to understand why the illness has affected them, what meaning it holds within their personal biography and how it can be integrated into a broader existential and social context. Mike Bury [8] highlights that illness constitutes a biographical disruption—a break in the expected course of life that threatens the coherence of personal identity. In response to this crisis, individuals are prompted to reconstruct their life story in an attempt at narrative repair, aimed at restoring a sense of continuity and comprehensibility of the experience. This process is inherently reflective and meaning-oriented: Individuals ask why the event occurred, what it means to them and how it can be explained. The stories people tell themselves and others not only stem from lived experience but are also profoundly shaped by the cultural, social and moral contexts in which they are embedded. Arthur Frank [9], through his theoretical elaboration based on his own experience with chronic illness, has emphasized how illness narratives are essential for coping with the existential dissonance that illness brings. He distinguishes three fundamental narrative types: the restitution narrative, which expresses hope for recovery; the chaos narrative, which conveys despair and a loss of control; and the quest narrative, which sees illness as an opportunity for personal transformation and the reorientation of values. In this latter form, narrative becomes a healing tool, in the sense of reorganizing the self and reconnecting with others. The centrality of narrative also emerges in contrast to the dominant biomedical model, often criticized for excluding the patient's lived experience. Bury refers to this as a "crisis of biomedical narratives" [8], driven by the growing prevalence of chronic illnesses, the medicalization of everyday life, the rise of alternative medicine and the spread of holistic approaches. In this context, patient narratives, once silenced by a paternalistic medical model, have gained new relevance as legitimate forms of knowledge and interpretation of illness. However, some criticisms, among them those directed at Frank, warn against an excessive idealization of illness's transformative potential, which risks slipping into a moralistic or spiritual rhetoric. Not all experiences of illness lead to existential rebirth; pain and loss may remain unassimilable. Nevertheless, the epistemological and existential value of narrative remains clear: It is a fundamental device through which ill individuals articulate the meaning of their experiences, negotiate their identities and reestablish a meaningful connection with the social world.

5.5 Focus Group with Students of the First Course "The Complexity of the Pharmacist-Patient Relationship: Towards a Pedagogy of Care"

A focus group was conducted as a conclusion to the educational journey undertaken with the students who attended the course "The Complexity of the Pharmacist-Patient Relationship: Towards a Pedagogy of Care" addressing the main themes explored throughout the course. The role of the pharmacist has undergone a profound transformation in recent years, especially following the COVID-19 pandemic and the recent reform that has made the degree in pharmacy a qualifying credential, evolving from a technical figure to a fully recognized healthcare professional. The pandemic marked a turning point: Pharmacists became an immediate point of reference for the public, providing concrete support not only through the dispensing of medications but also by offering essential health services, such as swab testing, vaccinations and the measurement of vital parameters. In this context, the pharmacist has assumed an active role in health promotion, gaining the trust of patients while also strengthening professional confidence and awareness of their competencies. The introduction of the qualifying degree has further enhanced the value of the profession, enabling graduates to enter the workforce directly and take on responsibilities from the outset. This change, however, entails the need to acquire both technical and relational skills during the university training process, increasingly emphasizing the integration of scientific knowledge with communication abilities. Topics such as empathy, effective communication, active listening and relational management have become fundamental in the education of the contemporary pharmacist. The ability to communicate clearly and understandably, adapting language to the patient's cultural and educational background, is crucial not only for ensuring therapeutic adherence but also for building a lasting relationship of trust. Within this evolving landscape, the pharmacist also assumes an educational role, countering health misinformation and promoting preventive behaviours and healthy lifestyles. The ethics of care, thus, becomes a guiding principle: caring for the patient as a person, rather than merely addressing the illness, means acting with empathy, honesty and a genuine orientation towards the well-being of others, rejecting purely commercial logic and consistently prioritizing the patient's health. The pharmacist is called to respond effectively to emergency situations and patient fragility, developing tools such as interdisciplinary collaboration, decision-making clarity, adaptability and narrative medicine, which allows for the understanding of patients' lived experiences. In parallel with these professional skills, the importance of self-care emerges as an essential condition for providing effective assistance. The pharmacist must maintain a balance between professional responsibilities and personal well-being, nurturing opportunities for reflection, physical activity and social connection in order to prevent burnout and remain empathetic and present. Lastly, digital transformation and artificial intelligence (AI) are redefining the operational framework of the profession. While AI offers the potential to improve work organization and access to information, it cannot replace the empathy, clinical judgement and human connection that remain at the core of the pharmacist-patient relationship. In a continuously evolving healthcare system, the pharmacist of the future will increasingly serve as a bridge between technology and humanity.

S.L.: In your opinion, how has the role of the pharmacist changed in recent years, especially after COVID and the reform that made the degree qualifying?

A.R.: In recent years, especially after the pandemic, which involved us all around the world, we can say that the pharmacist now has a more central and active role in the healthcare system. So, they are no longer seen—although this had started even before the pandemic—as just a simple dispenser of medicines, but rather as a healthcare professional who can offer consultations and provide direct support to patients. I would say that pharmacies have become true healthcare environments offering services that go well beyond just dispensing drugs. Just think about the vaccinations or all those paths defined as a "pharmacy of services", a mix of technical skills combined with the relational skills we've developed over the years. I think this, and I also believe the shift to the qualifying degree is crucial because it has helped enhance professionalism. We enter this world directly, but this implies that we must acquire both technical and relational skills already before and during our degree course. That time previously used between graduation and the state exam to gain these skills is now part of the degree itself, which is positive, but also requires stronger competencies.

E.B.: I think the role of the pharmacist, especially during COVID, became very important, because pharmacists became essential from every point of view. And also, the fact that the system changed and the degree became qualifying means that once we graduate, we can enter the workforce more quickly and take on the responsibility of being a pharmacist right away. That's what I think.

S.L.: So, during COVID, the pharmacist became more important, taking on a role comparable to other healthcare professionals, right?

E.B.: Yes, like a healthcare professional. Because during COVID, inside the pharmacy, you could get tested, have your blood oxygen level measured and more. With the qualifying degree, we can immediately enter the workforce, which is better than before when you had to take the state exam and only then enter the job market.

F.B.: Surely, during COVID, as Eleonora was saying, the pharmacist took on a fundamental role in society, being among the first to be in contact with patients, in addition to hospitals and testing centres. I think after COVID, trust in pharmacists really grew. The pharmacist gained more confidence in their abilities, but, above all, patients developed greater trust in the pharmacist—not just during COVID but even for advice beyond that.

S.L.: So, you're saying the pharmacist earned the patient's trust because they were out there on the front lines during a difficult time but also that they gained confidence in themselves. So, in some way, there was also recognition of your professional figure, which maybe before was a bit more overshadowed compared to other healthcare professions?

S.L.: Do you think the contents of the course, like communication, empathy, social influence and all the other topics we covered, will be useful in your future profession?

S. D.C.: Yes, I think the contents we covered in the course will be very useful for my future profession. We know well that being a pharmacist doesn't just mean dispensing medicines but also interacting daily with people who are often in fragile physical or emotional states. The relationship with patients who turn to the pharmacist in times of need requires an empathetic approach from the healthcare professional. Being empathetic helps establish a relationship of trust, increasing the likelihood that the patient will follow the correct instructions. Empathy is also key to understanding the real needs of patients, especially those facing chronic illnesses. To truly understand these needs, one must also master clear and comprehensible communication: This is fundamental for effectively explaining how to take medicines, highlighting possible side effects and answering patients' questions in simple terms. Effective dialogue helps reduce the risk of errors on both sides. A key skill is adapting your language depending on the patient's level of understanding, which is crucial to ensuring safety and adherence to prescribed therapies. Especially in recent years, with the explosion of online medical misinformation and harmful lifestyle advice, the pharmacist has taken on an important role in promoting healthy behaviours and debunking the many absurd claims people encounter on the web. Convincing someone to follow a proper therapy or change harmful habits requires a mix of persuasive skills, authority and tact that only professionals like us can offer.

N.F.: Yes, those are fundamental topics that are useful in any kind of training or job, in any work environment. So, definitely not only in the workplace, but in life in general—dealing with people is essential.

G.B.V.: In my opinion, communication and everything covered in the course are very important, because communication and empathy are key to building trust with patients, especially in delicate situations, to overcome the resistance that patients may have. Someone may not open up right away, and effective communication helps the pharmacist understand how to support them. It made me think of the book we had to read for our presentation, which talks precisely about the importance of building a relationship with the patient to be as efficient and effective as possible.

S.L.: Not everyone is ready to begin a therapeutic or care path, maybe because they're not ready to face their illness.

G.B.V.: Especially when the illness is serious, it might not be immediate.

G.P.: In one of the books we read for the course, it said that dialogue is the foundation of the relationship between pharmacist and patient because it's an exchange that happens between two people, thanks to words. Through this, the pharmacist can make the patient feel closer and even feel some compassion for them. The pharmacist plays an important role for the patient; they must be empathetic and recognize the patient as a person, a unique individual.

S.L.: Right, we've said it many times in the course: consider the patient as a person, not just as their illness, right?

C.P.: In my opinion, pharmacists—and healthcare workers in general—are increasingly involved in public health education campaigns. For us, this was the first real course where we talked about these topics, but I think in the future, once we start working, we'll need to take more courses like this. There's a growing public awareness, for example, on topics like adherence to therapy or disease prevention. We've also talked about that, and I think it reflects how the pharmacist's role has changed. Today, they've become a key figure for community well-being, not just someone who dispenses medicines.

S.L.: Yes, you said a key figure for the community, not just someone who hands out drugs.

C.P.: But really, for the well-being of the community, the population.

S.L.: How would you define the concept of care ethics within your professional role? We didn't go too deeply into the theme of ethics in the course—so, just ethics as a value, not as a historical or philosophical concept. What does "care" mean in the pharmacist's role?

M.R.: For me, care ethics means putting the patient's well-being at the centre of everything—not just caring for the illness, but for the person. This can only be done through empathy—being able to recognize the patient's emotions and teaching them how to manage those emotions. Ethics also means rejecting any behaviour that could harm the patient's health, like recommending a product just for profit.

G.R.: For me, care ethics is important in the pharmacist's role because empathy is crucial. The pharmacist must be empathetic to build a relationship—though still professional and confidential—with the customer, to get to know their history and give the best possible advice. They must act in the patient's best interest, not promote a product because it benefits them. A relationship of trust must be built, where the patient trusts the pharmacist.

S.L.: What tools should a pharmacist have to deal with difficult or emergency situations with particularly fragile patients?

J.M.: For me, the first thing is communication with colleagues. When dealing with fragile patients, we need to give them more attention and personal presence. So, communication, attention and understanding. Always have your tools ready and show empathy and listening—but, at the same time, also stay detached and rational when making decisions in emergencies.

S.D.: Communication skills are very important. We need to explain complex concepts in simple ways, adapting to the patient's level of understanding. If it's someone we know and who's knowledgeable, we can use technical terms. But otherwise, we should keep it simple. We also need to listen actively and recognize emotional or psychological needs that might come with the patient's issue. And we should collaborate with other pharmacists or the doctors who prescribed something. If it's a particularly fragile patient, maybe even with social workers.

S.L.: So, also build a bit of a network with other professionals?

S.D.: Yes, especially for pharmacists in small towns, where you know the regular patients. If you know someone is elderly and alone and relies on social services, it's helpful to connect with others to create a more supportive environment that encourages the patient to follow their therapy and not abandon it.

C.M.: I'd add that this brings us back to something we talked about during our presentation on narrative medicine: building a real relationship with the patient, especially if they are in a fragile situation. Or, like in class, we discussed people of different religions or customs—you need to know how to communicate with them. For example, how a man should approach a woman from another culture. Sometimes we take things for granted, but clarity is essential. Narrative medicine should be central to all healthcare professions. Also, in emergencies, you have to stay calm and avoid burnout, which we've talked about a lot. Don't let your emotions take over; stay clear-headed to truly help.

S.L.: How important is self-care, and what can each of us do to promote it?

J.M.: Self-care is fundamental. As we said in class, the pharmacist needs to feel good themselves to help others and give the right advice. Otherwise, their work becomes mechanical and rushed. So, it's important to reflect, take time for yourself, do sports, have fun and do things that make you feel good.

S.L.: Right, also to disconnect a bit?

J.M.: Yes. Our job, as passionate as we may be, will always push us to think more about others. So, self-care must start from within, listen to yourself, take time for reflection.

V.M.: For me, self-care means personal well-being, feeling good with yourself. In one of the books we read, there was a comparison between the pharmacist-patient and therapist-client relationship. The patient turns to a healthcare expert to clear their mind. If the pharmacist is filled with negative thoughts, they can't truly offer empathy or build trust with the patient.

S.L.: How do you think artificial intelligence will change the role of the pharmacist, and in what ways?

G.M.: AI is transforming healthcare in many ways, and pharmacists are no exception. It makes the profession more efficient but also requires pharmacists to evolve their skills. It can help offer more precise consultations, giving pharmacists fast access to clinical studies, guidelines and scientific updates. But this doesn't replace the human side of the professional.

S.D.C.: AI will have a major impact, changing many daily tasks and expanding responsibilities. Many repetitive tasks, such as inventory management, prescriptions, drug interaction checks, will be automated. This will allow more time for consultations and patient interaction. AI tools could suggest personalized dosages or alternative treatments based on the patient's profile. With digital tools, pharmacists could even remotely monitor therapy adherence and intervene if needed.

A.P.: Today, AI is transforming every profession. For pharmacists, I don't think it will ever fully replace them. Even if we use tools like ChatGPT, we don't get the human response we'd get from a real professional. So, yes, AI will influence the pharmacist's role, but I don't think we'll ever lose that human, empathetic and understanding element that comes from speaking face to face.[5]

5.6 Practice Time

1. What is meant by narrative pharmacy?
2. The experts interviewed mention the expression "teach-back". What does it mean?
3. What are rural pharmacies in Italy, and why are they important?
4. What changes with the reform of the qualifying degree course in pharmacy?
5. Can you describe the main topics involved in the focus group with students?

References

1. Law (Decreto Interministeriale) n. 651, 5-7-2022 "Laurea Magistrale a ciclo unico abilitante alla professione di Farmacista – Classe LM-13" (Based on articles 1 and 3 Law 8 November 2021, n. 163). Available from: https://www.mur.gov.it/it/atti-e-normativa/decreto-interministeriale-n-651-del-5-7-2022.

[5] Focus group with the students of the course "The Complexity of the Pharmacist-Patient Relationship: Towards a Pedagogy of Care", University of Siena, 24 January 2025.

2. Zigmond AS, Snaith RP. The hospital anxiety and depression scale. Acta Psychiatr Scand. 1983;67(6):361–70.
3. Scala D, Polvani S, Faggiano ME. Farmacisti del Servizio Sanitario Nazionale e COVID-19: le storie raccontano la professione ed il professionista. GIFAC. 2020;34(4):186–93.
4. Lopatriello S, Bellante L, Consiglio A, Lacaita MV, Faggiano ME, Scala D. Analisi narrativa di una indagine conoscitiva sull'argomento: Io e il Team. GIFAC. 2024;38(2–3):75–84.
5. Faggiano ME, Scala D. Farmacia narrativa come strumento di formazione e ricerca: uno studio pilota. GIFaC. 2020;34(2):55–61.
6. Scala D, Menditto E, Caruso G, Monetti VM, Orlando V, Guerriero F, Buonomo G, Caruso D, D'Avino M. Are you more concerned about or relieved by medicines? An explorative randomized study of the impact of telephone counselling by pharmacists on patient' beliefs regarding medicines and blood pressure control. Patient Educ Couns. 2018;101(4):679–86.
7. Bissell p, Ryan K, Morecroft C. Narratives about illness and medication: a neglected theme/new methodology within pharmacy practice research. Part I: conceptual framework. Pharm World Sci. 2006;28(2):54–60.
8. Bury M. Illness narratives: fact or fiction? Sociol Health Illn. 2001;23(3):263–85.
9. Frank AW. The wounded storyteller. Chicago: University of Chicago Press; 1995.

Chapter 6
Medical Humanities

6.1 Introduction

The reflection on the relationship between Eastern (including traditional and natural) medicine and Western evidence-based medicine (EBM) reveals, beyond apparent divergences, a set of analogies and possibilities for integration. Eastern and natural medicine, with its emphasis on harmony among body, mind and environment, appears to contrast with the Western biomedical model, founded on experimentation and the measurability of clinical outcomes. However, a closer examination shows how these two perspectives can be seen as complementary: the former oriented towards the individual's holistic well-being, the latter towards scientific precision and methodological rigor. The emergence of narrative medicine (NM) and, in parallel, narrative pharmacy (NP) in recent decades has opened new avenues for unifying these approaches. Listening to the patient's narrative allows the integration of the dimension of disease, traditionally central in Western medicine, with that of caring for the person, more typical of Eastern sensibilities. The patient's illness narrative, understood not only as a biological event but also as a relational experience, restores the centrality of the subject and creates space for more inclusive forms of care. According to some scholars [1–3], several practices typical of Eastern medicine exhibit affinities with Western practices, suggesting that the gap between the two models is not insuperable but rather the result of a relatively recent separation linked to the evolution of modern science. Nowadays, the task of NM and NP could be to rebuild a common ground in which scientific precision does not exclude but rather enriches listening and relational engagement. In this framework, care does not stop at disease control but extends to understanding the person in their entirety, achieving a synthesis between evidence and experience, body and word.

S. Leoncini, *The Relationship between Pharmacists and Patients*, New Paradigms in Healthcare, https://doi.org/10.1007/978-3-032-21249-8_6

6.2 Medical Humanities, Narrative Medicine and Narrative Pharmacy

Orpheus and Eurydice

Hymen, called by the voice of Orpheus, departed, and, dressed in his saffron robes, made his way through the vast skies to the Ciconian coast: but in vain. He was present at Orpheus's marriage, true, but he did not speak the usual words, display a joyful expression, or bring good luck. The torch, too, that he held, sputtered continually, with tear-provoking fumes, and no amount of shaking contrived to light it properly. The result was worse than any omens. While the newly wedded bride, Eurydice, was walking through the grass, with a crowd of naiads as her companions, she was killed, by a bite on her ankle, from a snake, sheltering there. When Thracian Orpheus, the poet of Rhodope, had mourned for her, greatly, in the upper world, he dared to go down to Styx, through the gate of Taenarus, also, to see if he might not move the dead.

Through the weightless throng, and the ghosts that had received proper burial, he came to Persephone, and the lord of the shadows, he who rules the joyless kingdom. Then striking the lyre-strings to accompany his words, he sang: "O gods of this world, placed below the earth, to which, all, who are created mortal, descend; if you allow me, and it is lawful, to set aside the fictions of idle tongues, and speak the truth, I have not come here to see dark Tartarus, nor to bind Cerberus, Medusa's child, with his three necks, and snaky hair. My wife is the cause of my journey. A viper, she trod on, diffused its venom into her body, and robbed her of her best years. I longed to be able to accept it, and I do not say I have not tried: Love won.

He is a god well known in the world above, though I do not know if that is so here: though I imagine him to be here, as well, and if the story of that rape in ancient times is not a lie, you also were wedded by Amor. I beg you, by these fearful places, by this immense abyss, and the silence of your vast realms, reverse Eurydice's swift death. All things are destined to be yours, and though we delay a while, sooner or later, we hasten home. Here we are all bound, this is our final abode, and you hold the longest reign over the human race. Eurydice, too, will be yours to command, when she has lived out her fair span of years, to maturity. I ask this benefit as a gift; but, if the fates refuse my wife this kindness, I am determined not to return: you can delight in both our deaths.

The bloodless spirits wept as he spoke, accompanying his words with the music. Tantalus did not reach for the ever-retreating water: Ixion's wheel was stilled: the vultures did not pluck at Tityus's liver: the Belides, the daughters of Danaüs, left their water jars: and you, Sisyphus, perched there, on your rock. Then they say, for the first time, the faces of the Furies were wet with tears, won over by his song: the king of the deep, and his royal bride, could not bear to refuse his prayer, and called for Eurydice.

She was among the recent ghosts, and walked haltingly from her wound. The poet of Rhodope received her, and, at the same time, accepted this condition, that he must not turn his eyes behind him, until he emerged from the vale of Avernus, or the gift would be null and void.

They took the upward path, through the still silence, steep and dark, shadowy with dense fog, drawing near to the threshold of the upper world. Afraid she was no longer there, and eager to see her, the lover turned his eyes. In an instant she dropped back, and he, unhappy man, stretching out his arms to hold her and be held, clutched at nothing but the receding air. Dying a second time, now, there was no complaint to her husband (what, then, could she complain of, except that she had been loved?). She spoke a last "farewell" that, now, scarcely reached his ears, and turned again towards that same place.

Stunned by the double loss of his wife, Orpheus was like that coward who saw Cerberus, the three-headed dog, chained by the central neck, and whose fear vanished with his nature, as stone transformed his body. Or like Olenos, and you, his Lethaea, too proud of your

> beauty: he wished to be charged with your crime, and seem guilty himself: once wedded hearts, you are now rocks set on moist Mount Ida.
>
> Orpheus wished and prayed, in vain, to cross the Styx again, but the ferryman fended him off. Still, for seven days, he sat there by the shore, neglecting himself and not taking nourishment. Sorrow, troubled thought, and tears were his food. He took himself to lofty Mount Rhodope, and Haemus, swept by the winds, complaining that the gods of Erebus were cruel.
>
> Three times the sun had ended the year, in watery Pisces, and Orpheus had abstained from the love of women, either because things ended badly for him, or because he had sworn to do so. Yet, many felt a desire to be joined with the poet, and many grieved at rejection. Indeed, he was the first of the Thracian people to transfer his love to young boys, and enjoy their brief springtime, and early flowering, this side of manhood. ([4] Bk X pp. 1–85).

This myth allows us to reflect on the power of love, on two souls bound together despite their separation between the world of the living and the realm of the dead and despite their differences. At the same time, it serves as a metaphor for human fragility, bearing witness to the fear of what is unknown and dreaded. The myth of Orpheus and Eurydice is one of the most significant narratives of classical tradition, for it embodies universal themes such as love, loss and the bond between life and death. Orpheus, the poet whose music could enchant men, animals and even the gods, represents the power of art and the spoken word, capable of transcending the boundaries of the earthly realm. His descent into the Underworld in an attempt to bring Eurydice back to life symbolizes humanity's longing to challenge destiny and the ultimate limit of mortal existence. Yet, his premature glance back at his beloved, condemning her to vanish forever, reveals the vulnerability and impotence of human beings in the face of death's mystery and the transience of existence. In this sense, the myth assumes a profound meaning: Love and art can illuminate human experience, but they cannot erase the pain and separation inherent to life. This myth also encapsulates the contradictions of human existence: perpetually poised between life and death, joy and suffering, hatred and love, sameness and difference.

6.2.1 Narrative Medicine

Maria Giulia Marini describes NM in her 2016 volume, *Narrative Medicine: Bridging the Gap Between Evidence-Based Care and Medical Humanities*, as "a bridge, or rather, a multiplicity of bridges, between clinical care and humanitas" [5] achieved through the use of mythology, literature, metaphor and scientific rigor: an approach capable of reuniting the fragmented domains of medical practice. Marini further proposes that NM may be applied as a genuine "scientific instrument", valuable both in patient care and the training of caregivers. Particularly intriguing is the analogy she draws between the relationship of EBM and narrative-based medicine and the turbulent yet passionate bond between Petruchio and Katherina, protagonists of Shakespeare's *The Taming of the Shrew* (1594) [5]. Their story is that of two lovers who, though profoundly different, strive to preserve their identities while ultimately reaching a state of harmony. Following their marriage, through quarrels and reconciliations, this peculiar form of concord grows ever stronger, forging a seemingly perfect couple, an allegory of the reconciliation of two paradigms that initially appear irreconcilable.

The term "evidence-based medicine" was coined, after years of research, by Gordon Guyatt and his team at McMaster University in Hamilton, Canada [6]. It designates a form of medicine grounded in evidence and demonstrable efficacy, understood as information that is both up-to-date and methodologically validated in the medical literature, i.e. through the results of studies establishing with scientific certainty the usefulness of a given treatment [7]. At the heart of this practice lies scientific data, which guide clinical decision-making. Within this framework, the patient does not actively participate in the therapeutic process but is regarded as the recipient of treatments supported by high-quality evidence. Illness is, thus, conceptualized as disease, an organic dysfunction stemming from a deviation in biological processes, with attention focused on causal pathways and the bodily effects of medical interventions.

Yet, the physician also undertakes a process of decoding and interpretation, akin to the paraphrasing of a poem, an act that no two readers would perform identically. The physician must interpret the patient's lived experience of illness, the problems reported by the patient, the findings of clinical examination and the results yielded by diagnostic technologies [8, 9]. An evidence-based framework does not, therefore, exclude empathic listening to the patient, nor the therapeutic use of the patient's own narratives of illness, which place lived experience at the centre of the healing process. The integration of EBM and narrative-based medicine, thus, aims at more comprehensive, personalized and effective clinical interventions, by harnessing the strengths of both. Multiple currents and approaches can be identified within NM itself. One of the most widely cited international definitions was elaborated by Rita Charon, foremost proponent of the humanistic-narratological approach, internist and professor of clinical medicine at Columbia University, New York, in her seminal volume *Narrative Medicine: Honoring the Stories of Illness* [10].

> We may call the narrative that medicine practiced with the competence to recognize, absorb, interpret, and be moved by the stories of illness. [...] Thanks to narrative medicine, one can more accurately identify illness, transmit knowledge and respect, collaborate humbly with colleagues, and accompany the patient, together with the family, through suffering. More ethical and effective care can be offered. This field gradually emerged from the confluence of various sources: the humanities, narratology, research on the physician–patient relationship ... It constitutes a concrete form of knowledge, which helps to understand not only the experience of patients, but also that of healthcare professionals themselves [10, p. 1]

At the core of the medical humanities lies NM, which conceives of illness not merely as a biological event but as a subjective experience and a story to be told. Narrative, thus, becomes a clinical tool, capable of enhancing communication, personalizing care and strengthening the therapeutic relationship. Listening to the patient means grasping fear, hope, perception of illness and its impact on daily life; conversely, narrating as a professional fosters reflection, prevents burnout and enables the rediscovery of the deeper motivations underpinning care [9]. The medical humanities constitute an interdisciplinary field uniting medicine with the humanities, history, philosophy, sociology, anthropology, ethics, literature and the arts, with the aim of restoring the human being to the centre of the care process. This approach seeks to "humanize" healthcare, moving beyond a solely scientific-technological understanding of illness and embracing the individual in their complexity: body, emotions, history, values and social context [11]. Although modern medicine tends towards increasing specialization and technical analysis, the medical humanities do not aspire to replace EBM but rather to integrate it, offering qualitative tools, such as narrative, to understand the experience of illness from both the patient's and the healthcare professional's perspective [12].

6.2.2 Narrative Pharmacy

The concept of narrative also extends to the pharmaceutical domain, giving rise to NP. Within this perspective, the pharmacist is not merely a dispenser of medicines but a trusted point of reference for health, with a crucial role in listening and counselling. Exploring the patient's history, taking into account their life context and fears, can enhance therapeutic adherence, strengthen the pharmacist-patient relationship and provide valuable insights into the real-world use of medications in daily life. Communication between patients and pharmacists constitutes a critical and delicate juncture within pharmaceutical practice. Misunderstandings, ambiguities and failures in mutual comprehension can easily lead to patient frustration, diminished trust in healthcare systems and, most importantly, reduced adherence to prescribed therapeutic regimens. While traditional strategies for improving communication, such as clinical guidelines, standardized checklists and increasingly sophisticated digital tools, undoubtedly play a valuable role, they often prove insufficient when confronted with the complexity of real-life encounters. Many patient-pharmacist interactions resist rigid standardization, as they frequently involve ambiguous, emotionally charged or highly individualized situations that require not only technical accuracy but also interpretive sensitivity. In this regard, the introduction of narrative methods, which have already acquired significant recognition and legitimacy within the fields of NM and the broader domain of the medical humanities, appears as a particularly promising innovation for enriching pharmaceutical practice. The concept of narrative competence refers to the healthcare professional's ability to read, interpret and critically analyse patients' stories as if they were texts, examining not only their explicit content but also their underlying structure, contextual framing, use of metaphor and strategic omissions. Through this interpretive process, pharmacists can gain access to clinically relevant information while simultaneously acknowledging the unique and often deeply personal experiences of illness that patients bring with them. Such an approach fosters a more nuanced, humanized and ethically attentive understanding of patients' lived realities. Educational research in related disciplines has consistently demonstrated that exposure to patients' illness narratives enhances students' sensitivity towards the needs and vulnerabilities of both patients and caregivers. These findings suggest that similar pedagogical strategies, if integrated within pharmaceutical training, could exert a transformative effect on professional formation. By cultivating attentiveness to narrative dimensions, future pharmacists may become better equipped to balance biomedical rigor with empathetic responsiveness, thereby developing a more holistic professional identity. A particularly illustrative case frequently cited in scholarly discussions [13] involves a 65-year-old male patient diagnosed with breast cancer, who approached his pharmacist with an apparently straightforward request: the purchase of apricot kernels as a possible therapeutic remedy. At first glance, this inquiry could be interpreted merely as a matter of product availability. However, a more attentive and narrative-sensitive reading of the encounter reveals a far more profound dimension. The patient's request was not only an attempt to obtain a specific substance but also an expression of his desire to sustain hope, reclaim a sense of agency over his illness and assert an active role within the therapeutic journey. The pharmacist's attentive listening and open-ended questioning enabled the emergence of meanings that extended beyond the biomedical dimension. The apricot kernels, while scientifically unsubstantiated as an effective treatment, carried a symbolic value for the patient: They represented a fragile yet powerful "opening" towards the possibility of healing. By recognizing this symbolic layer, the pharmacist was able to address the patient's existential concerns while simultaneously safeguarding clinical safety. The subsequent critical response, grounded in reliable scientific evidence, offered reassurance regarding the inefficacy and potential risks of the remedy requested, yet did so without dismissing or invalidating the patient's emotional investments. This episode demonstrates how the careful reception and interpretation of patient narratives can generate a dialogical space, where biomedical knowledge and personal meaning are not mutually exclusive but mutually enriching. In such a space, the pharmacist assumes the role of not only a technical expert but also an interlocutor, who sustains the therapeutic relationship through trust, empathy and interpretive competence. From this example, one can discern the broader professional implications of narrative practice for pharmacy. Narrative methods may serve as practical tools that enable pharmacists to (1) enhance the uniqueness of cases, (2) recognize implicit and metaphorical communication, (3) increase patient safety and satisfaction and (4) improve professional gratification. From this perspective, the systematic inclusion of training in narrative skills in pharmaceutical curricula and professional development programmes is proposed. The experience of NM demonstrates that a narrative approach, far from being dispersive, can reduce the risk of misunderstandings and make counselling more effective, ethical and patient-centred. Narration, in fact, plays a fundamental role in everyday life, enabling individuals to articulate, share and transmit their lived experiences, personal memories and expectations for the future. This narrative capacity assumes a critical significance within the healthcare context as it becomes a key instrument for achieving a comprehensive and multidimensional understanding of the patient. Such an understanding can be articulated through three interrelated conceptual dimensions: the disease, referring to the clinically defined and biomedically measurable condition; the illness, denoting the subjective and personal experience of suffering; and the sickness, understood as the broader social and cultural framework in which illness manifests and is interpreted. Narrative medicine has emerged as a clinical and care-oriented methodology that seeks to integrate technological and scientific knowledge with the humanization of medical practice. By placing emphasis on stories and relationships, NM advocates for a genuinely patient-centred approach, in which biomedical expertise is balanced by attention to the human, ethical and relational aspects of care. Within this conceptual and methodological landscape, NP can be situated as a specific adaptation of NM, explicitly oriented towards the professional role of the pharmacist and the practices of pharmaceutical care. The NP is primarily concerned with listening to and interpreting the stories told by patients, as well as those shared among healthcare professionals. Through this attentiveness to narrative, NP fosters a more holistic and relational comprehension of care, thereby contributing to the humanization of pharmaceutical services. Crucially, NP also restores to pharmacists their full professional identity, acknowledging them not merely as technical experts in the dispensing of medications but as active and dialogical participants within the therapeutic journey. By adopting a narrative stance, pharmacists are recognized as professionals capable of engaging empathically and collaboratively with patients, colleagues and other healthcare figures. This orientation situates them as integral agents of care rather than peripheral technicians. At the same time, NP poses an identity challenge, particularly for pharmacists employed within national healthcare systems, where their professional role is often underappreciated, misunderstood or conflated with that of other health workers. The first systematic references to NP date back to the biennium 2006–2007, when a series of articles published in *Pharmacy World & Science* highlighted the relevance of narrative approaches in the management of pharmacological treatments, especially in relation to chronic conditions. In subsequent years, international research further expanded upon these early insights, exploring how narrative strategies could be effectively integrated into pharmacy practice as part of the broader paradigm of patient-centred care. Scholars have emphasized that narrative approaches, when combined with the rigor of EBM, have the potential to improve not only the quality and safety of care but also patients' adherence to long-term treatment regimens. In particular, the use of narrative interviews has proven especially valuable: Such methods enable the collection of qualitative data with methodological rigor while also producing materials that can be meaningfully integrated with quantitative measures. The result is a more complete and multidimensional understanding of how illness and treatment impact the daily lives of patients.

From a methodological standpoint, NP frequently employs grounded theory as a framework for the coding and analysis of narratives [14]. This approach makes it possible to generate conceptual categories directly from the characteristics of the data and the affinities that emerge among them, rather than imposing preconceived theoretical structures. Narratives may assume different orientations within this analytic scheme: They can be disease-centred, focusing primarily on the clinical and technical aspects of pharmaceutical practice, or illness-centred, engaging more directly with the emotional, symbolic and relational dimensions of patient experience. Attending to both modalities allows healthcare professionals to interpret care dynamics in a richer and more nuanced manner. In doing so, it becomes possible to design diagnostic, clinical and therapeutic pathways that move beyond the mere management of pathological conditions and, instead, encompass the full experiential and social complexity of illness.

In conclusion, NP can be regarded as a significant contribution to the broader field of narrative healthcare, an umbrella concept that underscores the importance of storytelling as a means of connection, comprehension and humanization in all domains of health practice. The pharmacist's role is not only enriched by integrating pharmaceutical practice with narrative approaches but also repositioned at the centre of the care process. This integration strengthens the pharmacist's identity as a healthcare professional, enhances the quality of assistance provided and fosters a model of healthcare that is more participatory, empathetic and authentically patient-centred.

6.3 The Ethical Dimension of Care After the COVID-19 Pandemic

The care paradigm represents a fundamental approach in the context of research that entails profound attention to the well-being and dignity of the individuals involved, both as participants and subjects of study. Keeping this paradigm in mind means not only engaging in rigorous scientific research but also ensuring that research processes are ethical, responsible and sensitive to the needs and experiences of individuals. Adopting a care approach fosters a research environment that encourages mutual respect, solidarity and the awareness of the social and personal implications of discoveries. In an era where research can have a significant impact on people's lives, it is essential that researchers consider care a central component of their work, ensuring that every phase of the process, from planning to publishing results, respects principles of justice, empathy and social responsibility. Ethical responsibility in research is a fundamental issue to reflect on, closely linked to the meaning of caring practice. Knowledge of care is based on practice, a practice acquired by comparing specific cases and reflecting on them. Guiding ideas are those constructed experientially on the basis of ongoing comparative reflection on cases; as Martha Nussbaum [15] emphasizes, it is important to combine attention to the case in its singularity, having a sensitive perception of the particular, while referring to general principles through which one can question one's own thinking, even if no general principle can capture the complexity of reality. Central to this reflection is also Amartya Sen's theory of capabilities [16]. It is, therefore, necessary to develop a theory grounded in care, both in ethics and politics. In order to develop this theory, it is necessary to recognize that every individual, in both life stages marked by dependence and those in which independence increases, requires care, and, therefore, care must play a central role in the formation of ethical and political theories [17]. Indeed, there is no true ethics of care, but it is important to delve more deeply into the culture of care: It is a practice whose essence must be sought in the various ways of relating to others, including the learner, the person receiving care and the child. Care is guided by emotionally charged modes of thought. Therefore, an important issue to address is understanding the framework within which good care practices operate and, consequently, good research practices that take into account the emotional sphere of the research subjects. The framework within which care practices operate is constituted by ethical direction: We can conduct educational research with nurses, teachers, educators, caregivers and legal and educational officials. What emerges from this research is the goal of promoting well-being, experiencing this need as a necessity and helping others in their search for what constitutes a good life for them. Care is not an ethic, but an ethically informed practice, founded on principles such as conceiving ethics, questioning the quality of a good life and conceiving care as an action driven by the desire to promote the very need for a good quality of life [18]. Those who care seek to act within the realm of what is good, promoting the well-being of others. The three directions indicated by Luigina Mortari [19] in which the essence of the ethics of care lies are:

- Taking responsibility: From an Arendtian perspective [20], in which human beings cannot avoid acting it, is necessary to intervene by overcoming resistance to promptly engaging in a caring relationship, maintaining a distant proximity [21].
- Having respect: Without respect, there can be no good care, as Aristotle said: “Disrespect is the result of an opinion about something that seems worthless” ([22] Ret., II,1 p. 1378).
- Acting altruistically: Engaging in care means giving of one’s time and physical, emotional and cognitive energy, expanding the boundaries of the self [23].

We can conclude that within a research process, as in a care process, we know what we are offering, but we cannot predict the results we will obtain. The self, in fact, is encapsulated in the English term “serendipity”, which leads us to perceive the gift as external to the logic of the market.

The COVID-19 pandemic has posed a profound crisis in terms of not only health but also ethics and society, highlighting the structural and relational limitations of contemporary healthcare systems. One of the most significant effects has been the deterioration of public trust in healthcare institutions. As Tyler Evans observes [24], “the real public health emergency is the loss of trust”, a phenomenon fuelled by often contradictory communications and a widespread perception of inefficiency in managing the global crisis. This distrust has fostered the emergence of autonomous health management practices, including self-medication and the use of home remedies, which, in some contexts, have reached a prevalence between 7.14 and 88.3% [25]. Irene Kretchy and colleagues [26] document how “the use of home remedies for the prevention and treatment of COVID-19 symptoms represents a global trend towards autonomous health practices”, a phenomenon that reflects not only limited access to health services but also the need for personal agency in managing one’s own health. This scenario raises a fundamental ethical question: The excessive medicalization of everyday life, combined with clinical practice in which patients are insufficiently listened to, makes it essential to recognize the value of individual narratives. Telling one's story as a patient, thus, becomes a therapeutic and political act: It allows one to reclaim experiences often marginalized by biomedical logic and establish a more authentic dialogue with care. Jonathan McFarland [27], reflecting on the pandemic in the collection *Health Humanities for Quality of Care in Times of COVID-19*, suggests that contact with nature during lockdown reactivated profound therapeutic dimensions: "being in tune with the birdsong" [28] allowed him to rediscover a connection with the profound humanity of care. This example highlights how the ecological and humanist approach to medicine integrates narrative, listening and the environment, contributing to building a more empathetic, sustainable and profoundly human healthcare system. In conclusion, the pandemic has highlighted the urgent need to rethink the relationship between patient and healthcare professional, promoting transparent and empathetic communication and encouraging the active participation of citizens. The ethical dimension of care cannot ignore the valorization of individual stories, the centrality of listening and the awareness that health and well-being emerge from a balance between science, the environment and humanity.

6.4 Oriental Medicine, Homeopathy, Naturopathy and Phytotherapy

The landscape of so-called "alternative" or "complementary" medicine, an umbrella term that is often reductive, encompassing millennia-old disciplines such as Oriental medicine and more modern practices such as homeopathy, naturopathy and phytotherapy, represents a profound and radical challenge to the dominant scientific paradigm. It is not merely a different set of therapeutic tools but a veritable epistemological leap, a distinct way of conceptualizing life, illness, health and the relationship between humans and nature. This alternative perspective finds powerful expression in the writings and practices of authors such as Masanobu Fukuoka [29], for natural farming (a related philosophical system); Samuel Hahnemann [30], the founding father of homeopathy; and Maurice Mességué, a celebrated herbalist and a bridge to the general public, whose works, though popular in tone, are rooted in a profoundly philosophical naturopathy and phytotherapy [31]. The fundamental point of divergence, identifiable in both Hahnemann and the philosophical matrix of Oriental medicine, is the transcendence of the mechanistic-causal model. Conventional allopathic medicine, an heir to Descartes and Claude Bernard, tends to localize disease in a specific organ or pathogen, seeking to eliminate the symptom as if it were an enemy to be defeated. By contrast, for Hahnemann, as set forth in his *Organon der rationellen Heilkunde* (*Organon of the Healing Art*), the symptom is not the disease itself but the language through which the perturbed "vital force" (*dynamis*) attempts to react and communicate its imbalance [32]. The approach, therefore, is not to suppress the symptom (which, for Hahnemann, would only drive the disease into deeper layers of the organism, in a process termed "suppression", believed to be the origin of more serious chronic diseases) but to listen to it, meticulously catalogue it and find a substance that, in a healthy subject, can produce that same set of symptoms (*similia similibus curentur*, let like be cured by like). The homeopathic preparation, through successive dilutions and dynamizations (succussions), no longer acts on a biochemical-material level but on an energetic-informational one, stimulating the self-healing response of the vital force itself. This is a seismic shift in perspective: from waging war on disease to stimulating health. This concept of a "vital force" has an extraordinarily close counterpart in the concept of "ki" (or "qi") in Oriental medicine. This system was further developed and interpreted for the West by thinkers such as Michio Kushi, who, building on the work of George Ohsawa, articulated a comprehensive macrobiotic philosophy [33]. Kushi posited that health and disease are primarily determined by the quality of one's diet and lifestyle, which directly influence the balance of yin and yang energies within the body. In this model, health is the free and harmonious flow of ki through a network of channels called meridians. Disease is precisely a blockage, an excess or a deficiency of this flow. The therapist's task (through acupuncture, moxibustion, manual practices or dietary prescriptions) is to restore the dynamic balance between yin and yang, the two complementary polarities that govern the universe and, as a microcosm, the human body. Diagnosis, through pulse reading, observation of the tongue and general appearance, is, thus, holistic: It does not seek a specific bacterium or an altered blood value but assesses the overall energetic state of the individual. In this tradition, there is no separation between mind and body or between emotion and organ (anger is linked to the liver, worry to the spleen, fear to the kidneys). Healing, therefore, inevitably involves the entire person in their psychophysical unity.

It is precisely in this space of interconnection between humans and nature, between vital force and the power of plants, that the figure of Maurice Mességué is masterfully situated. If Hahnemann systematized the law of similars and thinkers like Kushi explained the principles of energetic balance, Mességué was the romantic and passionate standard-bearer of phytotherapy, understood not as the mere pharmacological use of active principles in plants but as a sacred art of dialogue with the "green force". This vision finds a robust scientific and philosophical parallel in the work of Jean Valnet, a French physician and pioneer of aromatherapy and phytotherapy [34]. Valnet argued rigorously for the therapeutic efficacy of plants based on their scientifically identifiable biochemical properties, effectively bridging the empirical wisdom of herbalism with the demands of modern science. He maintained that essential oils and plant extracts possess powerful antiseptic, antiviral and regenerative properties that act directly on the organism. Similar to Mességué, but from a more clinical perspective, Valnet saw plants not as simple vehicles for isolated compounds but as complex living entities whose synergistic components (the "totum") work in concert to restore health. Mességué, the son of a Pyrenean "herbal healer", always insisted that his practice was not medicine but a "lifestyle hygiene cure" based on the power of wild plants. In his writings, plants are not mere containers of useful molecules; they are living entities, charged with an intelligence and a vital energy (that concept again!) that can be transferred to humans. His phytotherapy is deeply naturopathic: The ultimate goal is not to treat a specific pathology but to purify the organism, to "cleanse the terrain", an expression also dear to naturopathy, to allow the body to heal itself. Mességué's detoxifying treatments, based on plants such as elderberry, birch and dandelion, aim to drain the emunctory organs (liver, kidneys, intestines, skin), freeing the body from the toxins that obstruct the free flow of life. In this, his vision connects both to the homeopathic principle of non-suppression (to drain rather than suppress) and to Oriental medicine (to unblock the flow of ki). Finally, naturopathy emerges as the practical and philosophical synthesis of all these contributions. While drawing from all these disciplines, the modern naturopath (following a tradition founded by figures such as Kneipp or Lust) acts primarily as a health educator. Their main tool is not a drug but advice on a lifestyle: natural nutrition (often based on vitalistic and detoxifying principles), physical exercise, stress management and hydrotherapy. Their role is to identify and remove obstacles to health (*causa tollens*), supporting the *vis medicatrix naturae*, the healing force of nature inherent in every individual. This concept is the perfect Latin counterpart to Hahnemann's "vital force", the "ki" of Oriental medicine and the vital energy described by Mességué and Valnet.

In conclusion, although homeopathy, Oriental medicine, phytotherapy and naturopathy use different languages and techniques, from infinitesimal dilutions to acupuncture needles and from detoxifying herbal teas to dietary regimens, they are united by a holistic and vitalistic vision of the human being. They see disease as the end product of a deeper imbalance, whether a disturbance of the *dynamis*, a blockage of ki or an accumulation of toxins. Therapy, therefore, is not an act of aggression against an external enemy but a work of rebalancing, stimulation and support for the organism's innate self-healing capabilities. The authors cited, Hahnemann with his systematic rigour, the macrobiotic philosophers like Kushi with their dietary principles, Mességué with his passion for the plant world and Valnet with his scientific validation of plant essences, remind us that medicine can also be an art, a respectful dialogue with the forces of nature and a profound trust in the intelligence of life that inhabits every organism. It is a perspective that, beyond the inevitable scientific controversies that accompany it, invites greater individual responsibility for one's own health and a reconnection with the rhythms and remedies of the natural world.

6.5 Practice Time

1. What is narrative medicine?
2. What is narrative pharmacy?
3. What has changed regarding the theme of the ethics of care after COVID?
4. How does "alternative medicine" distinguish a different way of conceptualizing life, illness, health, and the relationship between humans and nature compared to EBM?

References

1. Nutton V. Ancient medicine. London: Routledge; 2005.
2. Goody J. The Eurasian miracle. Cambridge, UK: Polity Press; 2010.
3. Hadot P. La philosophie comme manière de vivre. Paris: Albin Michel; 2001.
4. Ovid. The Metamorphoses, Book X (version by Kline AS). University of Virginia Library; [cited year not provided]. Available from: https://ovid.lib.virginia.edu
5. Marini MG. Narrative medicine: bridging the gap between evidence-based care and medical humanities. Cham: Springer; 2016.
6. Guyatt GH. Evidence-based medicine. American College of Physicians Journal Club, Editorial, 1991: A-16. Available from: https://www.jameslindlibrary.org/guyatt-gh-1991/
7. Straus SE, Glasziou P, Richardson WS, Haynes RB. Evidence-based medicine: how to practice and teach EBM. 5th ed. Amsterdam: Elsevier; 2018.
8. Greenhalgh T. What is narrative based medicine? BMJ. 1999;318(7178):323–5.
9. Greenhalgh T, Hurwitz B. Narrative based medicine: dialogue and discourse in clinical practice. London: BMJ Books; 1999.
10. Charon R. Narrative medicine: honoring the stories of illness. New York: Oxford University Press; 2006.
11. Evans HM. Medical humanities: stranger at the gate. Med Humanit. 2007;33(2):85–90.
12. Jones DS, Wear D, Friedman LD, editors. Health humanities reader. New Brunswick: Rutgers University Press; 2014.
13. Naß J, Banerjee M, Efferth T, Wohlmann A. Pharmaceutical care as narrative practice? Rethinking patient-centered care through a pharmacist's perspective. Int J Clin Pharm. 2016;38:1346–9.
14. De Fina M, Consiglio A, Monzillo J, Lacaita MV, Centola R, Lopatriello S, et al. Farmacia narrativa: un "nuovo" approccio alla cura. GIFaC. 2025;39(2):124–31.
15. Nussbaum MC. Creating capabilities: the human development approach. Cambridge, MA: Belknap Press of Harvard University Press; 2011.
16. Sen AK. Development as freedom. Oxford: Oxford University Press; 2001.
17. Noddings N. Starting at home: caring and social policy. Berkeley: University of California Press; 2002.
18. Tronto JC. Moral boundaries: a political argument for an ethic of care. New York: Routledge; 1993.
19. Mortari L. La pratica dell'aver cura. Milan: Pearson; 2022.
20. Arendt H. The human condition. 2nd ed. Chicago: University of Chicago Press; 1958.
21. Zambrano M. El pensamiento vivo de Séneca. Madrid: Ediciones Siruela; 1994.
22. Aristotle. Retorica. Milan: Arnoldo Mondadori Editore; 1996.
23. Derrida J. Donner le temps. Paris: Éditions Galilée; 1991.
24. Evans T. Commentary: the real public health emergency is loss of trust. My Journal Courier [Internet] 2025 [cited 20 Aug. 2025]. Available from: https://www.myjournalcourier.com/opinion/article/the-real-health-emergency-loss-trust-tyler-20818240.php
25. Al-Hanawi MK, Angawi K, Alshareef N, Qattan AMN, Helmy HZ, Abudawood Y, et al. A systematic review of self-medication practice during the COVID-19 pandemic. Front Public Health. 2021;9:1041695.
26. Kretchy IA, Osei AD, Asiedu E. Use of home remedies for the treatment and prevention of COVID-19: an integrative review. J Complement Integr Med. 2022;19(1):1–9.
27. Marini MG, McFarland J, editors. Health humanities for quality of care in times of COVID-19. Berlin: Springer Nature; 2022.
28. Lovatt S. Birdsong in a time of silence. London: Particular Books; 2021.
29. Fukuoka M. The one-straw revolution. New York: NYRC Classics; 2009.

30. Stöteler ECW. Hahnemann's homopathy: the classification of treatment of diseases according to Dr. Samuel Hahnemann. Doldersweg: Success BV;2020.
31. Mességué M. Health secrets of plants and herbs. New York: HarperCollins; 1979.
32. Hahnemann S. Organon der rationellen Heilkunde. Dresden: Arnoldischen Buhhandlung; 1810.
33. Kushi M. Natural healing through macrobiotics. Tokyo: Japan Publications; 1979.
34. Valnet J. The practice of aromatherapy. Saffron Walden: C. W. Daniel Co. Ltd.; 1982.

Chapter 7
The Future of Pharmacists

7.1 Introduction

The digital transformation of healthcare is redefining the operational boundaries of pharmaceutical practice, with online pharmacies and AI emerging as key drivers of this transition. E-pharmacies have evolved over the past decade from niche digital marketplaces to a global industry exceeding one hundred billion USD in value, offering unprecedented convenience, accessibility and integration with digital health ecosystems. This expansion has been accompanied by the rise of telepharmacy services, which extend pharmaceutical care to remote and underserved populations through digital platforms. At the same time, AI has introduced a new paradigm in medicine and pharmacology, enabling data-driven diagnostics, drug discovery and personalized treatment planning. However, while these innovations promise enhanced efficiency and patient access, they also pose significant ethical, regulatory and professional challenges. Concerns regarding counterfeit medicines, data privacy and the erosion of the pharmacist-patient relationship underscore the need for a careful balance between technological advancement and human-centred care. Moreover, the integration of AI into pharmacy practice requires rigorous oversight to ensure accuracy, transparency and accountability, while preserving the empathetic and relational dimensions of care that technology cannot replicate. This chapter critically examines the transformative role of online pharmacies and AI within contemporary pharmaceutical practice, exploring their implications for regulation, professional identity, patient safety and the future training of healthcare professionals. It argues that sustaining a patient-centred ethos, grounded in ethical responsibility, empathy and collaborative practice, will be essential for harnessing digital innovation without compromising the integrity of care delivery.

S. Leoncini, *The Relationship between Pharmacists and Patients*, New Paradigms in Healthcare, https://doi.org/10.1007/978-3-032-21249-8_7

7.2 Pharmacy and Artificial Intelligence: Online Pharmacies

Online pharmacies have undergone a rapid global expansion in recent years, reshaping the way patients and consumers access pharmaceutical products. The global e-pharmacy market has already surpassed one hundred billion USD in value and is projected to grow several-fold in the coming decade, driven by convenience, competitive pricing and increasing integration with digital health systems. Parallel to this expansion, telepharmacy services, defined as the remote provision of pharmaceutical care through video consultations, telephone or online platforms, have gained particular relevance in reaching underserved populations, such as those living in rural or remote areas. These services now constitute an emerging subsector of the global pharmaceutical market, offering not only medication dispensing but also patient counselling, medication management and adherence support. Among the key actors in this field is Amazon, which entered the pharmaceutical sector through the acquisition of PillPack and the subsequent launch of Amazon Pharmacy. Amazon has positioned itself as a disruptive force in the industry by combining large-scale logistics, Prime membership benefits and competitive subscription models, such as RxPass. Its services allow patients to order medications online with fast or even same-day delivery, integrate their insurance information and benefit from pharmacist consultations. Strategic partnerships with pharmaceutical companies, such as collaborations with Eli Lilly, further extend Amazon's role in the direct-to-consumer model for prescription medicines. This expansion highlights the growing convergence between global technology platforms and healthcare delivery. Nevertheless, the growth of online pharmacies brings important risks and challenges. Regulatory authorities have long warned against the proliferation of illegal or unregulated e-pharmacies, many of which distribute substandard or counterfeit medicines. This poses a serious public health concern, particularly in low- and middle-income countries where supply chains may already be fragile. Furthermore, the convenience and anonymity of digital platforms risk diminishing the traditional therapeutic relationship between pharmacists and patients. The pharmacist has historically played a central role in not only dispensing medications but also offering professional advice, reassurance and individualized care. As digital channels dominate, this relational dimension risks being eroded, potentially undermining the holistic value of pharmacy practice. Looking forward, the future of e-pharmacy will probably be defined by the development of integrated omnichannel systems, blending digital convenience with in-person care. Technological advances in AI, automation, blockchain and wearable devices may allow more personalized and data-driven pharmaceutical services. Yet the sustainability of this model depends on effective international regulation, robust safeguards for drug quality, patient privacy and the preservation of professional standards. Telepharmacy, when properly implemented, offers opportunities to extend access without sacrificing quality, but it must be coupled with training and support for pharmacists to ensure that digital care retains its human dimension. David Healy argues in "Pharmageddon" [1] that the excessive reliance on technological systems within healthcare professions risks undermining the very capacity of physicians, pharmacists and nurses to exert a positive therapeutic influence on their patients. The challenge is to maintain a balance between caring for the patient and searching for a cure. This equilibrium is particularly vital in circumstances where a definitive cure is not possible, and the healing relationship itself, rooted in empathy, trust and professional presence, becomes a crucial therapeutic resource.

7.3 Digital Transformation in Pharmacy and Medicine: Online Pharmacies and Artificial Intelligence

The digital transformation has profoundly impacted both the pharmaceutical and medical sectors, giving rise to new models of healthcare delivery and innovation. Among these, online pharmacies (e-pharmacies) and AI in medicine represent two key developments that are reshaping how patients access care and medical and pharmaceutical professionals operate. Online pharmacies have emerged as a significant reconfiguration of traditional medicine distribution channels. They offer notable advantages globally, including improved access, convenience and discretion for patients, particularly for those with limited mobility or living in remote areas. E-pharmacies can enhance treatment adherence while reducing logistical and privacy-related barriers by enabling home-based access to medications. However, the development of online pharmacies varies widely and is closely linked to national and regional regulatory frameworks, creating a fragmented landscape with substantial disparities in safety and quality control. Online pharmacies in highly regulated regions, such as the United States and the European Union, adhere to strict protocols. In the United States, accreditation programmes, such as the Verified Internet Pharmacy Practice Sites run by the National Association of Boards of Pharmacy, certify legitimate operators [2]. Similarly, the European Union has implemented a common mandatory logo that verifies a pharmacy's authorization in the national registry of the corresponding member state and ensures that prescription-only medications are dispensed only with valid prescriptions. By contrast, low- and middle-income countries often experience weaker or inconsistently enforced regulation, facilitating the proliferation of illicit operators. This unregulated market poses serious risks, including the distribution of counterfeit drugs, which may contain incorrect dosages, toxic ingredients or lack active ingredients entirely, threatening public health. Additional concerns include breaches of patient data privacy and the absence of professional pharmaceutical consultation, which is crucial to prevent adverse drug interactions. Consequently, while authorized online pharmacies can complement traditional healthcare services, consumers bear significant responsibility for identifying legitimate providers and ensuring proper consultation with qualified healthcare professionals. Artificial intelligence is another transformative technology in healthcare, with applications spanning disease diagnosis, drug discovery and treatment optimization. Artificial intelligence systems analyse large datasets, recognize patterns and generate predictions with speed and precision exceeding human capabilities. Utilizing advanced mathematical models, such as machine learning and deep learning, AI can learn from provided examples to make increasingly accurate decisions, making it a revolutionary tool in both medicine and pharmacology. In clinical practice, AI enhances diagnostic accuracy and supports treatment planning. It can analyse medical imaging, electronic health records and scientific literature to detect anomalies, predict disease risk and enable early interventions. Surgical procedures can also be assisted by AI, improving precision and reducing invasiveness, complications and recovery time. Furthermore, AI facilitates remote patient monitoring and personalized therapy management. In pharmacology, AI accelerates the discovery of new drugs by analysing vast databases of chemical compounds and biological data. It identifies promising molecules, expedites experimental validation and even suggests repurposing existing medications for new therapeutic applications. Artificial intelligence, for instance, has contributed to the development of DSP-1181 for obsessive-compulsive disorder and INS018_055 for idiopathic pulmonary fibrosis, as well as identifying new antibiotics against resistant bacteria and repurposing raloxifene as a potential therapy for COVID-19. Despite these advances, AI does not replace human clinicians. Medical decision-making relies on experience, clinical context and patient interaction, elements that AI cannot replicate. Moreover, empathy, essential for establishing trust and tailoring treatment, remains beyond AI's capabilities. The integration of AI into healthcare introduces several challenges. Privacy concerns are paramount, as AI processes large volumes of sensitive patient data. Poorly trained AI systems, based on biased or non-representative datasets, risk generating inaccurate clinical recommendations. The legal responsibility for AI-generated errors is also unresolved in many jurisdictions. Trust in AI depends on its transparency, reliability and interpretability, allowing healthcare professionals to validate its outputs and ensure patient safety. The future implementation of AI in medicine and pharmacology requires clear regulatory frameworks to safeguard data use, prevent diagnostic errors and define legal accountability. Human oversight remains essential to ensure that AI serves as a supportive tool, enhancing but not replacing medical expertise. The convergence of digital technologies in pharmacy and medicine, through online pharmacies and AI, represents a profound transformation in healthcare delivery and pharmaceutical innovation. Online pharmacies can increase access and convenience, particularly in underserved regions, while AI enhances diagnostic accuracy, therapeutic efficacy and drug discovery. Both developments require robust regulation, professional oversight and informed patient engagement to maximize benefits and mitigate risks. Healthcare systems can foster safer, more efficient and more personalized care by embracing these technologies responsibly, ultimately empowering both patients and healthcare professionals in an increasingly interconnected digital ecosystem.

7.4 How the Future of Pharmacists and Patients Will Change with Artificial Intelligence

While the pedagogy of care emphasizes human relationships and empathic listening, research on AI demonstrates its transformative potential across diverse domains. A 2022 study by the European Commission highlights fundamental elements to be considered when discussing the opportunities that AI offers for the cultural and creative sectors. The document, entitled Opportunities and Challenges of Artificial Intelligence Technologies for the Cultural and Creative Sectors [3], examines the challenges posed by AI and proposes possible actions for stakeholders and policymakers at both national and international levels, with the aim of promoting a culturally diverse European offer. The attention devoted by the European Commission suggests that, although scientific literature on the topic has multiplied in recent decades (a full review of this literature cannot be provided here due to limits of time and space), awareness of these issues is essential to prepare for an inevitable future that will impact multiple sectors, including education and healthcare. Francesco Lavanga and Maria Mancaniello [4] argue that the goal is to identify possible pedagogical responses to the digital age in order to safeguard and support individual development. Their hope is to offer insights that will stimulate reflection on how the roles of educators and trainers at every level will change and how such professional figures must prepare themselves for the profound transformations that our society is undergoing. At the same time, prominent scholars are reflecting on the implications of AI for the healthcare sector. Joachim Roski and colleagues [5] maintain that AI will increasingly serve as a support to physicians, rather than replacing them, assisting in complex tasks and reducing physical and cognitive fatigue among healthcare professionals. Although concerns persist regarding privacy and data regulation, AI can also facilitate faster access to information for citizens. An example is the Italian Electronic Health Record system, which has streamlined patient data consultation. Roski and colleagues further note that AI will likely offer significant benefits to vulnerable groups, such as older adults or individuals in situations of fragility and poverty, by improving access to care in resource-constrained contexts. From an educational perspective, however, recent research on educational and cultural poverty [6] reveals that this issue does not exclusively affect children from disadvantaged socio-economic backgrounds but cuts across all social classes. Nevertheless, it is particularly acute in complex urban contexts, such as peripheral areas, which can be seen as a metaphor for contemporary society itself—complex, contradictory and marked by blurred boundaries—where social phenomena are more pronounced and diffuse [7]. Starting from a realistic analysis of material, moral, cultural and educational deprivation that particularly affects younger generations, pedagogical research is urged to reflect on the relationship between education, schooling and poverty [7], also in connection with AI and digital technologies that, especially during the COVID-19 pandemic, have become an integral part of school life [8]. The United Nations Regional Information Centre noted in a 2023 report that the relationship between AI and economic as well as professional inequalities is at the centre of an intense global debate. According to the report, technological automation has contributed between 50 and 70% of the overall rise in economic inequality among social groups in the United States since the 1980s. The danger is that AI may reproduce and even amplify these inequalities across professional fields, the labour market and in the relationship between capital and labour. Yet the United Nations emphasizes that AI tools can also be used to enhance the skills of a wide range of workers, from manufacturing to office and creative work, as well as to strengthen democratic participation and civil society engagement. However, realizing such promises requires a significant reorganization of the ways in which AI is developed and applied. Enhancing professional skills and reinforcing democratic participation, thus, demand a structural rethinking of AI development and application. This perspective underscores the urgency of a critical approach to technological governance, aiming to balance innovation with social equity. The challenge lies in integrating AI within inclusive organizational models while avoiding new forms of exclusion or technocratic dependency [9]. Artificial intelligence plays an increasingly crucial role in contemporary society by optimizing complex processes, personalizing services and improving efficiency in fields such as healthcare, education and social assistance. It can support vulnerable individuals, such as the elderly and persons with disabilities, through predictive models and behavioural analytics, by offering adaptive solutions and continuous monitoring [10]. Its integration is now indispensable for ensuring equity, inclusion and sustainability, reducing socio-economic disparities and empowering vulnerable populations. Nevertheless, despite its ability to replicate cognitive processes and simulate complex interactions, AI cannot replace human empathy, which is rooted in subjective experience, emotional connection and authentic responses to unpredictable situations. While chatbots may imitate emotional language, they lack the phenomenological consciousness that guides compassion and contextual adaptation. Empathy requires a shared vulnerability that AI, lacking corporeality and intentionality, cannot experience. Its ideal role is, therefore, one of support, rather than substitution, within helping relationships.

7.5 Identity and Training for Online Life in Future Pharmacists

Reflections on identity, digital identity, media and social networks assume a central role in the contemporary context, characterized by the pervasive presence of digital technologies and the growing interconnection between online and offline life. Understanding how the construction of the self is influenced by digitally mediated interactions is essential for university students in pharmacy, who must develop critical, ethical and professional skills within complex and interconnected environments where they will increasingly interact with patients through digital channels. The process of digitalization does not merely consist in translating the analogue into the digital; rather, it represents a cultural, social and medial crossing of boundaries, where narrative and communicative forms are incessantly remediated. Drawing on Marshall McLuhan's insight [11] that "the content of a medium is always another medium", the concept of remediation, introduced in the 1990s by Jay Bolter and Richard Grusin [12], describes the phenomenon whereby one medium appropriates the techniques, forms and social meanings of other media, competing with or reshaping them in the name of the real. In this sense, a new medium remediates the previous one, preserving its positive features while simultaneously offering solutions to its shortcomings. In the specific case of the pharmacist-patient relationship, this implies that styles of reading and narration cannot remain unaffected by the continuous processes of remediation through which new (digital) media transform older analogue media. Some studies report that individuals in the Western world switch sources of information at least 27 times per hour, check their phones over 150 times a day and consume more than 34 gigabytes daily across multiple devices [13]. This data helps us understand how such dynamics have generated a practice of hyper attention while simultaneously lowering the threshold of tolerance for boredom. We are more easily distracted due to a paradoxical process: Hyperattention forces us to disperse, moving rapidly from one digital focus to another, perceiving meanings rather than interpreting them. Consequently, one shifts from skimming to skipping to browsing. Within this context, narrative forms have also been transformed, marked by the hyper-segmentation of space and time, fragmentation and multiplication of narrative linearity, dissolution of the author/reader distinction, continuous shifts between narrative levels and the reticular structure typical of hypertext. The spread of digital technologies and the pervasive diffusion of connectivity and networking practices form the premises for the emergence of a participatory and convergent culture based on the ideas of sharing and collective intelligence [14]. Charles Horton Cooley introduced the notion of the "looking-glass self" [15] in 1902, arguing that identity emerges through a relational process in which others' opinions and feedback function as mirrors for self-understanding. This process is amplified in today's digital age: Interactions on social media, content views and comments become powerful instruments that shape the self-perception and awareness of one's choices and behaviours, underlining the importance of critical and conscious authenticity. Complementary to this perspective is George Mead's work [16], which distinguishes between the "I" and the "Me". The "Me" represents the internalization of social norms, whereas the "I" embodies creativity and the capacity to innovate in interactions. For pharmacy students, this distinction translates into the need to balance the influence of the academic community, peers and professional references with their own critical initiative, both in digital interactions and face-to-face contexts. Online platforms extend the concept of the "generalized other", offering new spaces where social and professional norms are continuously articulated and negotiated. In this context, narration assumes a central role. Paul Ricœur [17] distinguishes between idem- and ipse-identity: The former concerns coherence and permanence, while the latter refers to the capacity for renewal and fidelity to oneself in the face of change. The construction of a coherent narrative allows students to integrate academic, professional and digital experiences, fostering a professional identity that is self-aware, adaptable to constantly evolving contexts yet internally consistent. The use of digital technologies also influences the representation of professional identity. Online platforms not only provide spaces for self-expression but also determine the conditions of visibility and interaction, thereby shaping reputation and professional relationships. Awareness of these dynamics is crucial for developing problem-solving skills and decision-making autonomy, both of which are essential in the training of future pharmacists. Digital competence constitutes an indispensable tool within educational contexts. The European Union [18] defined digital competence as the ability to use information technologies critically and responsibly for learning, working and communicating. This competence includes information literacy, collaboration, digital content creation, safety and problem-solving, integrating technical knowledge with civic and social awareness. Digital habits represent the practical expression of competencies, defining recurrent behaviours in the interaction with technologies [19]. Reflection on these habits enables university students to develop a conscious use of online platforms for both scientific research and professional communication, thereby fostering autonomy, critical thinking and ethical responsibility. According to "A Companion to Digital Ethics" [20], the ethical dimension of digital life is central: Awareness of the implications of technologies for identity construction, scientific data management and professional communication is fundamental. Students must acquire the capacity to navigate between opportunities and risks, using digital tools in an ethically responsible manner, to the benefit of their own training and the safety of the contexts in which they will operate. In summary, contemporary academic and professional life is immersed in a digital ecosystem that interweaves identity, competencies and habits. Understanding onlife dynamics, constructing coherent narratives and reflecting on digital practices are crucial components in the education of pharmacists, contributing to the formation of critical, ethical and self-aware professionals capable of operating in an increasingly interconnected scientific and social world.

7.6 Can We All Do Better?

One day, a one-year-old child was brought to the bustling surgical clinic in Nanded. On the parents' faces was that expression of fear, helplessness, and fervent hope that I had learned to recognize in overcrowded, under-resourced hospitals. The little boy lay in his mother's arms, alarmingly still, with his eyes open but showing no interest or engagement. His breathing was regular and relaxed, yet unnaturally fast, as if a pump inside him were running at the wrong speed. The mother described repeated, terrifyingly violent bouts of vomiting, the emesis splashing beyond the table. A doctor in the paediatric clinic had noticed an enlarged head, with a circumference visibly disproportionate to the small body, and made a provisional diagnosis confirmed by a skull X-ray: the child had severe hydrocephalus, a congenital condition in which normal brain drainage is blocked. Cerebral fluid accumulates slowly, progressively enlarging the skull but also compressing the brain to mitigate pressure. Without surgical intervention to provide the fluid a new exit from the skull and brain, brain damage worsens, progressing from vomiting to vision loss, drowsiness, coma, and ultimately death. However, if the surgery succeeds, the child could have a perfectly normal

> life. Therefore, the paediatricians had referred the parents and the child to the surgical department. Unfortunately, there were no neurosurgeons. Nor did the department have the necessary equipment for a neurosurgeon: no drill to make a hole in the skull, no sterile one-way shunt tube to divert the fluid from the brain under the skin to the abdominal cavity. The surgeons, however, did not want to let the child die this way. They explained to the father what kind of instrument was needed for the operation, and he managed to find a makeshift version at the local market for 1500 rupees, about thirty dollars. It wasn't perfect, the tube was too long and not sterile, but P. T. Jamdade, the chief surgeon, still agreed to operate. The child was taken to the operating room the following morning, my last day in Nanded, so I could witness the procedure. The tube was cut and sterilized in an autoclave. The anaesthetist put the child to sleep with a ketamine injection, an effective and inexpensive anaesthetic. A nurse shaved the right half of his head and disinfected him from head to pelvis with an iodine-based antiseptic. A young doctor placed sterile gauze around the surgical site. On a small tray under the single lamp, a nurse arranged the surgical instruments—silvery, shiny, and, to my eyes, wholly inadequate for the task. Jamdade had just a bit more than I would use to suture a small laceration. Nevertheless, he grabbed the scalpel and made an incision about three centimetres long. He took a haemostat— a common metal clamp similar to scissors that surgeons usually use to hold a small blood vessel or suture thread—and slowly wedged its tip into the child's exposed skull. At first, nothing happened. The tip kept slipping on the hard bone surface. But then it caught, and for fifteen long minutes Jamdade meticulously scraped until a tiny hole opened in the skull. He then worked to widen the opening, taking extreme care not to puncture the now-exposed brain. When the gap was large enough, he inserted one end of the tube into the space between the brain and skull, threading the other end under the skin of the neck and down towards the abdomen. Before placing the tube into the open abdominal cavity, however, he paused to observe the fluid as it drained from the brain through the new channel. It was clear and friendly, like water. Like perfection. Jamdade had not given up. And so, at least, that child would live [21]

In the final episode of the series "Adolescence" [22], Jamie, a 13-year-old boy, tells his parents that he has decided to plead guilty to the murder of a peer. The scene is set in the same room from which the narrative began, the room where the young boy was arrested at dawn by the police about a year earlier. The father, weeping and devastated by grief, sitting on his son's bed opposite his favourite stuffed animal, reflects on his own role, his possible shortcomings and the ways in which he might have prevented such an extreme act, at least tried to access that world confined within the locked bedroom. That room, a metaphor for an isolation that can take many forms, from the social withdrawal of hikikomori to the identity crises of incels, to more widespread expressions of distress, becomes the symbolic place where parenting is called upon to exercise its caregiving function. The issue of care as a relational paradigm emerges in the play "Wit" [23], Pulitzer Prize 1999, albeit differently from "Adolescence". The main character, a university professor suffering from terminal cancer, finds herself surrounded by doctors who prioritize a technical and scientific approach, neglecting the human and empathetic dimension of caregiving. It is only in her relationship with a nurse that she experiences a genuine form of closeness, based not on clinical expertise but on attention to the need for comfort, listening and presence. This element highlights a condition that unites seemingly distant situations: the sense of inadequacy that accompanies those who care [24]. The same tension arises in the case of a parent reflecting retrospectively on the impossibility or inability to access their child's inner world, as well as that of someone caring for a sick person and questioning whether they have done enough, or a doctor lacking the tools to perform an operation that could save a child's life. It is the awareness that care is never entirely sufficient, that there is always a margin of helplessness, an area of fragility beyond control, especially when there is no collaboration among the different figures involved, who need to work in synergy like the organs of a healthy, robust human body. This awareness, far from leading to paralysis, can become the core of an ethic of care that accepts limitations, acknowledges incompleteness and, precisely because of this, strengthens the commitment to remain present, improve, try to do better and strive to do the best to save others' lives. Whether in the parent-child relationship or in that between caregiver and care recipient, care, thus, appears as an act measured not by absolute effectiveness but by the quality of the relationship and the ability not to abandon the other. The concept of Gross National Happiness (GNH), conceived by the King of Bhutan, Jigme Singye Wangchuck, in the 1970s, is much more than just an alternative economic indicator; it is a state philosophy that radically challenges Western notions of progress and well-being. While the predominant development model equates a nation's success with gross domestic profit growth and material consumption, GNH proposes a holistic and pluralistic vision of happiness. It suggests that there is no single, universally valid idea of the "good life" but that it must be defined according to the cultural, social and environmental context of a community. The GNH acknowledges that fundamental rights and economic well-being (measured in the "Living Standards" domain) are necessary but insufficient conditions for collective happiness. True progress emerges from a dynamic balance between nine distinct but interconnected domains. These include health and education, but they give equal weight to factors often overlooked by Western metrics: community vitality, ecological resilience, psychological well-being, balanced time use, cultural diversity and resilience and good governance. In this way, Bhutan contests the cultural hegemony of Western development models. The GNH implies that a wealthy individual in a Western megacity might be considered "poor" or "not yet happy" according to the Bhutanese index if, despite having a high income, they suffer from loneliness (low community vitality), stress (poor time use) or live in a degraded environment (low ecological resilience). The index, in fact, methodically measures "sufficiency" in each of these aspects, classifying as "happy" only those who achieve a high level of balanced well-being in two-thirds of the indicators. The results of the latest 2022 report, which show an improvement in the index despite global economic adversity, demonstrate the resilience of this approach. The GNH does not reject material well-being, but relativizes it, placing it within a broader framework of shared values. It, thus, opposes the idea that happiness is a standardized, exportable commodity, proposing it instead as a contextual equilibrium that is multidimensional, and whose definition belongs to each society based on its own history and cultural and spiritual priorities. Choosing to dedicate oneself to a profession that truly inspires passion, even when it does not immediately guarantee financial reward, represents a commitment that transcends personal interest: It acknowledges that the value of our work is constructed through its connection to others. Erich Fromm observes [25] that love is not merely a feeling but a conscious act requiring attention, care and responsibility towards those around us; to love is to recognize the profound interconnection that binds our existence to that of every other person. In the context of pharmacy, this principle translates into how we relate to patients: actively listening, understanding their needs, responding with empathy and also listening to ourselves, our doubts and our insights. It is through this attentive engagement, this genuine connection, that the ability to perform our work with responsibility and dedication emerges. This spirit of dedication is vividly illustrated in the pages of Atul Gawande [26, 27]. The seemingly simple rule for physicians, always striving, always seeking something more without ever giving up, serves as a guiding principle for pharmacists as well: it is not enough to know medications or follow protocols; it is essential to cultivate curiosity, meticulous attention and the continuous desire to improve. Virginia Apgar's work [28], which revolutionized the assessment of newborn health through her meticulous attention, demonstrates how precise and mindful care can save lives and transform generations. Yet, as Gawande emphasizes, individual dedication alone is insufficient: Collaboration among colleagues, dialogue between healthcare providers and families, and the daily sharing of experiences and knowledge are fundamental to effective care. In other words, each individual's skill and commitment are amplified only when embedded within a network of relationships, where listening, respect and mutual responsibility become as essential as technical knowledge or practical experience. This logic manifests in the pharmacy setting through concrete actions: taking the time to understand patients, clearly explaining medication usage, jointly evaluating effects and alternatives and engaging in constructive dialogue with colleagues. Every small act of attention forms a chain of responsibility that enables continuous improvement. Just as the central question in medicine often concerns whether to invest in research or enhance existing care, in modern pharmacy, especially with the advent of digital technologies and online platforms, we must consider how to reconcile innovation with professional ethics: AI and online pharmacies are not ends in themselves, but tools that can enhance patient care, expand possibilities and improve service quality, provided the human dimension remains central. Pursuing work we love also involves accepting a tension: that between capitalism and love, between financial gain and dedication, between efficiency and care. Fromm teaches us that love entails responsibility and interconnection and that believing in it means believing in the possibility of authentic relationships in which everyone contributes to the common good. This principle is not abstract: It manifests in daily actions, in every attention paid to a patient and in every constructive exchange with a colleague. As in Apgar's work and Gawande's observations, continuous improvement arises from careful observation, the analysis of outcomes and the humility to recognize what can be done better. Every choice, explanation or small piece of advice has a real impact in pharmacy: It saves time, prevents errors, enhances health and strengthens patient trust. Therefore, the pharmacist of the future, even while immersed in advanced technologies and digital platforms, must maintain a central focus on listening and caring. This requires courage: the courage to prioritize the patient, continually learn, collaborate without reservation and accept that perfection is never a static state but an ongoing journey. Only then can the pharmacy become a space where competence and humanity intersect, technical innovation harmonizes with ethical responsibility and daily practice becomes an act of love capable of generating real well-being and leaving a lasting mark on people's lives. In this interplay of passion, dedication and listening, of knowledge and interconnection, lies the key to not only performing our work well but also restoring to pharmacy, whether traditional or digital, its deepest meaning: being a place of care, trust and authentic human connection.

7.7 Practice Time

1. What are the pros and cons of an online pharmacy instead of a normal pharmacy?
2. How do you think that AI is going to contribute to digital transformation in pharmacy and medicine?
3. How will the future of pharmacists and patients change with AI?
4. Have you ever thought about doing better in your job?

References

1. Healy D. Pharmageddon. Berkeley: University of California Press; 2013.
2. National Association of Boards of Pharmacy. VIPPS: Verified Internet Pharmacy Practice Sites [Internet]. [cited 2025 Aug 23]. Available from: https://nabp.pharmacy/programs/vipps/
3. European Union. Opportunities and challenges of artificial intelligence technologies for the cultural and creative sectors. Luxembourg City: Publications Office of the European Union; 2022. [Online] Available from: https://op.europa.eu/en/publication-detail/-/publication/359880c1-a4dc-11ec-83e1-01aa75ed71a1/language-en
4. Lavanga F, Mancaniello M. Formazione dell'adolescente nella realtà estesa. La pedagogia dell'adolescenza nel tempo della realtà virtuale, dell'intelligenza artificiale e del metaverso. Padova: Libreriauniversitaria.it; 2022.
5. Roski J, Gillingham B, Juse E, Barr S, Sohn E, Sakarcan K. Implementing and scaling artificial intelligence solutions: considerations for policy makers and decision makers. [Internet] Health Affairs Blog 2018 Sep 17 [cited 2025 Apr 6]. Available from: https://www.healthaffairs.org/do/10.1377/hblog20180917.283077/full
6. Marone F. La speranza nella cura, la speranza per la cura. Lecce: Pensa MultiMedia; 2022.
7. Tolomelli A. Bologna: da centro a periferia del welfare educativo. Civitas Educationis Educ Polit Cult. 2016;5(1):61–81.
8. Di Bari C. Servizi educativi 0-6 e digitale, dopo la pandemia: riflessioni pedagogiche. SSFOJE. 2022;25(2):41–8.
9. Praetorius I. L'economia è cura. La riscoperta dell'ovvio. Naples: IOD; 2016.
10. Luxton DD, editor. Artificial intelligence in behavioral and mental health care. London: Elsevier Academic Press; 2016.
11. McLuhan M. Understanding media: the extensions of man. Cambridge, MA: MIT Press; 1994.
12. Bolter JD, Grusin R. Remediation: understanding new media. Cambridge, MA: MIT Press; 1999.
13. Koji J, Shigeaki I, Satoshi N, Masaki T, Hiroki C, Norihiro S, et al. The neural basis of task switching changes with skill acquisition. Front Hum Neurosci. 2014;8:339–48.

14. Levy M, Gurevitch M. Defining media studies: reflections on the future of the field. Oxford: Oxford University Press; 1994.
15. Cooley CH. Human nature and the social order. New York: Scribner's; 1902.
16. Mead GH. Mind, self and society: from the standpoint of a social behaviorist. Chicago: University of Chicago Press; 1934.
17. Ricœur P. Oneself as another. Chicago: University of Chicago Press; 1992.
18. European Union. Recommendation of the European Parliament and of the council of 18 December 2006 on key competences for lifelong learning. Off J Eur Union. 2006;L394:10.
19. Varona-Gómez F, et al. Digital habits in contemporary contexts. Comput Human Behav. 2025;143:107600.
20. Floridi L, Taddeo M, editors. A companion to digital ethics. Hoboken: Wiley-Blackwell; 2025.
21. Gawande A. Better: a surgeon's notes on performance. New York: Metropolitan Books; 2007.
22. Barantini P. Adolescence. Netflix; 2025.
23. Edson M. Wit. London: Hern Nick; 1999.
24. Tronto JC. Moral boundaries. A political argument for an ethic of care. New York: Routledge; 1993.
25. Fromm E. The art of loving. New York: Harper & Row; 1956.
26. Gawande A. The checklist manifesto: how to get things right. New York: Metropolitan Books; 2009.
27. Gawande A. Being mortal: medicine and what matters in the end. New York: Metropolitan Books; 2014.
28. Apgar V. A proposal for a new method of evaluation of the newborn infant. Curr Res Anesth Analg. 1952;32(4):260–7.

MIX
Papier aus verantwortungsvollen Quellen
Paper from responsible sources
FSC® C105338

If you have any concerns about our products,
you can contact us on
ProductSafety@springernature.com

In case Publisher is established outside the EU,
the EU authorized representative is:
Springer Nature Customer Service Center GmbH
Europaplatz 3, 69115 Heidelberg, Germany

Printed by Libri Plureos GmbH
in Hamburg, Germany